突发公共卫生事件快速风险评估

Rapid Risk Assessment of Acute Public Health Events

主审　冯子健

主译　倪大新　金连梅

译者　涂文校　孟　玲　洪志恒　李雷雷
　　　曹　洋　张　甜　赵梦娇

U0391821

世界卫生组织

人民卫生出版社

Rapid Risk Assessment of Acute Public Health Events
《突发公共卫生事件快速风险评估》由世界卫生组织 2012 年出版。
© 世界卫生组织，2012 年
世界卫生组织总干事授予人民卫生出版社翻译和出版本书中文版的权利，
中文版由人民卫生出版社全权负责。

图书在版编目（CIP）数据

突发公共卫生事件快速风险评估 / WHO 主编；倪大新，
金连梅译. —北京：人民卫生出版社，2014
ISBN 978-7-117-19850-9

Ⅰ. ①突… Ⅱ. ①W… ②倪… ③金… Ⅲ. ①公共卫
生－突发事件－风险评价－中国 Ⅳ. ①R199.2

中国版本图书馆 CIP 数据核字（2014）第 233489 号

人卫社官网	www.pmph.com	出版物查询，在线购书
人卫医学网	www.ipmph.com	医学考试辅导，医学数据库服务，医学教育资源，大众健康资讯

版权所有，侵权必究！

突发公共卫生事件快速风险评估

主　　译：倪大新　金连梅
出版发行：人民卫生出版社（中继线 010-59780011）
地　　址：北京市朝阳区潘家园南里 19 号
邮　　编：100021
E - mail：pmph @ pmph.com
购书热线：010-59787592　010-59787584　010-65264830
印　　刷：北京盛通印刷股份有限公司
经　　销：新华书店
开　　本：710×1000　1/16　印张：5
字　　数：95 千字
版　　次：2015 年 12 月第 1 版　2017 年 8 月第 1 版第 3 次印刷
标准书号：ISBN 978-7-117-19850-9/R·19851
定　　价：29.00 元

打击盗版举报电话：010-59787491　E-mail：WQ @ pmph.com
（凡属印装质量问题请与本社市场营销中心联系退换）

目　录

引　言

　　本手册用于指导世界卫生组织（以下简称 WHO）成员国对各种形式危害引起的突发公共卫生风险进行快速评估。主要使用对象包括国家健康保护部门、《国际卫生条例》（International Health Regulations，IHR）国家归口单位与 WHO 工作人员。本手册还可供参与多学科风险评估的临床、现场流行病学、兽医、化学及食品安全等领域专家参考使用。

　　本手册通过指导系统地开展事件识别、风险评估及对利益相关者和公众开展风险沟通，对突发公共卫生事件做出快速且经得起质询的决策。

　　本手册是对下列风险评估指南的补充：

- 《世界卫生组织人类健康风险评估工具包：化学危害》[1]
- 《风险分析在食品标准问题中的应用》[2]（1995 年 3 月 13～17 日瑞士日内瓦 FAO、WHO 联合专家咨询会）

　　风险评估已经逐渐成为突发公共卫生事件应对中的一项常规工作，希望读者能够提供宝贵改进建议及用于培训的实践案例。

目的

　　突发公共卫生事件的快速风险管理可减少或预防受累人群疾病的发生，并减轻其对社会和经济的负面影响。此外还有以下作用：

- 使决策更经得起质询
- 控制措施更加适宜且及时
- 工作沟通更加有效
- 风险沟通更加有效
- 优化应急准备

决策经得起质询

　　风险评估时考虑并记录当时所有可用的相关信息。这一过程为决策提供支持和指导：

- 对哪些风险和控制措施进行了评估

---

[1]　http://www.who.int/ipcs/publications/methods/harmonization/toolkit.pdf

[2]　http://www.who.int/foodsafety/publications/micro/march1995/en/index.html

- 使用的评估方法
- 为什么认为它们重要
- 优先顺序

如果持续进行记录，则可以反映出事件发展过程中以下内容的变化：

- 评估的风险等级
- 推荐的控制措施
- 关键的决策和行动

根据风险评估的系统记录，对风险评估工作本身进行评价，确定今后风险评估和卫生事件响应工作需要改进之处。

控制措施及时适当

系统收集分析事件相关的危害、暴露及背景信息，有利于：

- 确定基于证据的控制措施；
- 比较控制措施的适宜性及可行性；
- 确保控制措施与公众健康风险水平相适应。

此外，事件发生过程中风险评估工作会持续开展，决策者可根据更新的相关信息及时调整控制措施。

工作沟通更为有效

使用通用的风险评估术语，可以极大提升参与事件评估和响应的机构内部上下级之间、部门之间以及和机构外部工作的沟通效率。

风险沟通更为有效

公众风险沟通的目的是向目标人群宣传建议个人和社区采取的预防、缓解措施。有效的风险沟通是在公众信任和同理心的基础上，及时、透明地分享所有相关信息。突发公共卫生事件风险评估可以确定关键的预防、缓解措施，为有效风险沟通提供依据。

优化应急准备

本手册侧重于突发公共卫生事件发生时的风险评估，同时也适用于应急准备工作，特别是季节性与周期性暴发事件的应急准备（如非洲每年的霍乱暴发疫情，美洲和亚洲地区的登革热季节性流行）。

在协助制定应急准备规划方面，风险评估可用于确定高危地区或高危人群、准备活动的优先性，并确定关键的政策和合作伙伴。

手册编写过程

2010 年 11 月，在日内瓦成立由 WHO 驻成员国代表处、区域办公室以及总部人员组成的手册编写工作组。包括：

- 公共卫生事件监测人员；
- 公共卫生事件风险评估人员，包括针对多类危害或专门针对食品安全、化学危害等领域的人员；
- 有经验的应急领导者；
- 有经验的风险评估培训人员。

此外动物卫生专家也参与了本手册的制定，WHO 风险沟通专家及 IHR 专家提供了建议。工作组人员名单与电话会议参与人员名单见附录 6。

相关术语

本手册中，突发公共卫生事件是所有暴发或是进展迅速，可能对人类健康造成负面影响，需要立即开展评估和应对的事件。包括尚未引起人类患病，但可能因暴露于受污染的食物、水、产品、环境或染疫动物而导致人类患病的情形。

不同学科对风险的定义不同。本手册中，风险是指在特定时期内，发生不良事件的可能性及其后果的严重性。不同学科和部门中使用的与公共卫生相关风险术语的比较详见附录 1。

不同学科对风险的定义存在差异有其历史原因。本手册针对需要多学科和多部门协作的突发公共卫生事件风险评估，所以制定术语时综合参考了多学科定义（详见附录 2）。

全危害策略与国际卫生条例

多年来，全危害策略应用于突发事件和灾害管理中，用于描述自然、技术或人为事件，这类事件发生后需要为了保护生命、财产、环境、公共健康或安全而采取行动，以减轻社会危害。

全危害策略适用于需要立即响应，可能由多个危害引起的公共卫生事件，包括自然、意外或人为释放的生物、化学和放射性危害，以及火灾、洪水、极端天气、火山爆发、地震及海啸等自然灾害。

为应对日趋频繁的国际旅行和贸易，有国际传播风险的新发或再发疾病以及化学物、毒物和放射物的威胁，IHR 于 2005 年进行了修订。IHR（2005）推进了全危害策略在公共卫生领域的应用。

IHR 要求各缔约国按照条例要求构建一系列监测和应对的核心能力，涵盖"对人类构成或可能构成严重危害的任何疾病或医学问题，无论其病因或来源如何"。

风险评估后，各成员国根据 IHR 中附件 2 的决策文件要求，决定是否需要将突发公共卫生事件向 WHO 正式通报。附件 2 的有效使用有赖于各国当局和 IHR 国家归口单位（National Focal Point，NFP）对其领土内发生的公共卫生事件开展风险评估。

按照 IHR 监测和应对核心能力的要求，各成员国应建立国家级（可能情况下，省及以下）的风险评估能力，该能力是预防、监测和响应系统不可分割的一部分。风险评估的组织和定位，根据各国国情可以是一个专门的小组，也可以作为现有预防、监测和响应系统中的一部分。

尽管各个成员国风险评估的组织和定位有所不同，WHO 及其成员国应采用一致的、结构化的方法对突发公共卫生事件进行风险评估。推荐的结构化风险评估步骤如下。

公共卫生事件的侦测及确认

WHO 所有成员国都建立了发现传染病暴发的监测系统。鉴于 IHR 重点强调加强此项核心能力建设的要求，多数成员国已将其监测系统扩大至包括其他危害导致的公共卫生事件。公共卫生事件监测系统包括：

● 指标监测：根据病例定义按照预先设定的指标常规收集疾病信息[1]（例如急性弛缓性麻痹病例的每周监测）。通常预先设定暴发阈值用于预警和响应。

● 事件监测：快速收集突发公共卫生事件关键信息。事件监测的信息来源包括各种官方与非官方途径，用以发现具有相似的临床症状和体征，但其临床表现与常见疾病不符的聚集性病例。官方信息来源包括国家政府当局和官方组织（如联合国系统）。非官方信息来源包括媒体、其他非官方的公共信息（如互联网站）以及公众报告。

指标监测和事件监测系统报告和预警的事件并不一定都是真实的，也不一定都具有重要的公共卫生意义。"假阳性"事件（即报告的事件不是真实的事件，或指标监测系统的报告数据已超过阈值，但不是真正的暴发疫情）的数量与监测系统的目的和设计有关，同时也与开展事件评估机构的层级有关。

制定的指导意见应可以协助工作人员对新监测到的事件进行筛检和评估（框1）。对事件进行筛检需要评估该事件可能造成的公共卫生风险，其原则与本手册中介绍的更加正式的风险评估原则相同。

框1 监测人员对监测信息筛检评估的示例

问题	回答
事件报告是否来自官方渠道（如当地疾病控制机构、医疗卫生机构、畜牧兽医部门、林业部门等）？	是□ 否□
事件报告是否来自多个独立的渠道（如公众、新闻媒体、医疗卫生工作者、畜牧兽医人员）？	是□ 否□
事件描述是否包括时间、地点和波及人员的具体信息（如参加某社区庆祝活动3天后有6人发病、2人死亡）？	是□ 否□
是否有病例临床表现描述（如7人因非典型性肺炎住院，其中2人死亡）？	是□ 否□
此前是否有类似事件报告（如同一时期，有相似的临床表现，受影响人群及地区分布相似）？	是□ 否□

注：表格中所列问题回答"是"的数量越多，所收集的信息是真实事件的可能性就越大

如果在事件发生早期被迅速识别，那么最初获得的信息可能是有限且非特异的。最初的筛检过程重在评估所获信息的可信度，以及所描述的事件是否对公共卫生具有潜在风险进而需要开展调查。事件报告的准确性可能也需要同时评估。事件的确认并不意味着它会给公众健康带来风险。某些事件对人类健康的影响很小或几乎没有，或可能与慢性病相关但不会带来紧急的公共卫生风险。因此，应根据最初的风险评估结果采取相应的行动措施（见表1）。

---

[1] 此处"疾病"一词使用引申义，包括症状的含义。

5

表1 事件分类与确认后采取行动举例

事件分类及确认结果	行动措施
事件被证实为虚假的谣言	结束关注该事件； 根据需要开展风险沟通和媒体沟通，使公众对该事件的风险有正确的认识（如关于天花的谣言）
事件属实但不是紧急的公共卫生风险	继续跟踪该事件，当获得进一步的事件信息时，开展风险评估； 根据需要开展风险沟通和媒体沟通，使公众对该事件的风险有正确的认识
事件属实且可能是紧急的公共卫生风险	开展全面的风险评估，并说明评估的可信水平； 向决策者提供建议，包括应采取的行动措施及各行动措施的优先顺序（例如推荐的控制措施、关键的沟通信息）； 当获得进一步的事件信息时，继续开展风险评估，并调整相应的决策建议。根据风险评估结果，不同级别机构采取的行动措施是不同的

风险评估介绍

风险评估是对事件信息进行收集、评估、记录并确定事件风险等级的系统过程，为减少突发公共卫生风险的不良后果提供行动依据。风险管理环（图1）包括：

● 风险评估：指危害评估、暴露评估、背景评估以及作为划分事件风险等级依据的风险水平描述；

● 确定可能的控制措施：针对受影响的人群及社会，考虑控制措施的效果、可行性及可能的不良影响，并确定措施的优先顺序；

● 对事件进展进行持续跟踪和评估；

● 开展有效沟通，以保证风险管理者、其他利益相关者和受影响的社区理解并支持所采取的控制措施；

● 在事件应对结束后开展评价，总结经验及教训。

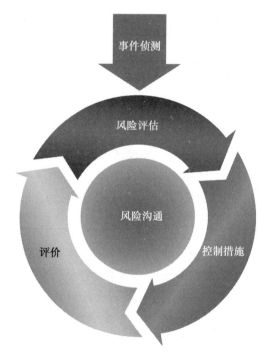

图1 风险管理环

公共卫生事件风险评估步骤

组建风险评估团队

当确认某一事件属实并认为该事件可能引发紧急的公共卫生风险时,就必须开展风险评估,确定其公共卫生影响。根据可用的信息的质量和完整程度,组建风险评估团队。确定风险评估团队专家的专业背景是往往被忽视却非常关键的环节。评估过程中,可能需要随时纳入新的专家(如毒理学、动物医学、食品卫生学、辐射防护等领域)。但是当存在以下情况时,在组建评估团队之初就需要包括上述专家:

- 不明原因危害
- 事件由传染性病原体引起的可能性小
- 事件涉及动物发病或死亡,和(或)疑似动物源性传染病
- 事件涉及食品安全或产品召回、化学物质、放射事故(不管是否有人类发病)

业务沟通和公众沟通是风险管理的重要组成部分。应在风险评估团队与风险沟通专家之间建立良好的协作机制。如果条件允许,风险评估时应邀请风险沟通专家加入。在风险管理过程中始终确保决策者和受影响人群之间有良好沟通,有助于提高控制措施的实施效果,尤其是公众需要在事件应对时做出行为改变的情况。

风险评估的质量很大程度上受风险评估团队的学识及专业水平的影响。事件发生地相关背景信息是风险评估的关键依据之一。突发公共卫生事件的风险等级取决于发生地的社会、经济、环境和政治背景以及当地医疗卫生水平(如临床和公共卫生服务)。对于某些危害,卫生部门和其他相关部门及机构(如负责动物源性疾病的动物卫生部门)之间的沟通协作机制也会影响事件的风险水平。因此组建风险评估团队时需考虑上述因素。

确定风险问题

风险评估团队应确定需要回答的主要风险问题,以助于界定风险评估范围、确保全面收集风险评估所需信息。同时,清晰明确的风险评估问题也有利于在风险评估时确定优先开展的行动。明确风险评估问题,可通过文献综述、流行病学调查、加强监测、专家咨询及科研来实现。

通常来说,风险问题围绕以下方面设立:

- 可能受影响的人群

- 暴露于危害的可能性
- 人群暴露于危害后产生不良后果的时间、原因及方式

风险评估团队提出的风险问题还受到下列因素的影响：

- 高危人群
- 开展风险评估的层级，如地方级、省级、国家级、国际（如跨境）或全球；
- 风险评估团队专业和机构背景，以及他们对于所评估事件的集体经验，如是已充分认识的疾病还是不明原因（如不明病原）公共卫生事件
- 决策者、其他利益相关者和社会对风险的可接受水平
- 事件发生过程中开展风险评估的时机
- 既往事件与类似情形的风险评估结果
- 国际社会等外部机构对事件的知晓情况和关注度

风险评估团队不用试图在事件发生之初就立刻回答所有的风险问题，应该首先确定需要立即解决的关键问题，一些不紧迫的问题可以留待以后解决或交给其他团队解决。

突发公共卫生事件中需要回答的首要问题是"事件的公共卫生风险是什么"（例如，在特定地点暴露于特定危害的风险是什么，或特定人群在特定时间的风险是什么）。

围绕上述问题，常常要回答：

- 如果不采取控制措施，暴露于危害的可能性有多大？
- 如果某事件发生，造成的公共卫生后果是什么？

风险问题可以基于一系列场景假设，如：

- 在现有情况下，事件发生的公共卫生风险是什么？
- 事件播散到某个大城市的公共卫生风险是什么？
- 事件影响多个地区（省份/州，国家）的公共卫生风险是什么？

其他基于不同场景的风险问题示例见表2。

表2　风险问题示例

事件	风险问题
1～2天内相邻的两个农场共52头猪死亡	该事件是否对人类健康造成风险？
出现聚集性HIV/AIDS患者突然治疗无效	造成此事件的原因是什么？如： - 继发感染 - 药物不合格（假药或药物过期导致效力下降） - 耐药 - 药物可及性（几名病人分服一人的药物或病人难以获得药物） - 病人治疗依从性

事件	风险问题
医务人员不明原因肺炎导致死亡	可能导致肺炎的原因？ 可能的公共卫生后果？
一个特定区域的难民营内发生霍乱，2人死亡，16例疑似病例	霍乱疫情进一步扩散的可能性？ 霍乱疫情进一步扩散的后果？
含有乙二醇的小儿止咳糖浆导致多名儿童聚集性死亡	该产品是否出口到国外，包括合法或走私方式？ 如果已出口国外后果如何？
某国家14个省中有一个省出现托儿所儿童的手足口病疫情暴发	在事件发生地区采取检疫措施对控制疾病传播的效果如何？ 在感染地区采取检疫措施将如何影响疾病的传播？ 在感染地区采取检疫措施的后果如何？

根据事件性质，风险评估团队需要确定后续风险评估的频度、各问题的优先性及每次风险评估的完成时限。两次风险评估之间的间隔将有助于确定应考虑风险问题的数量及内容。

开展风险评估

某一事件的风险水平取决于可能（或已知）的危害、暴露于危害的可能性以及事件发生的背景。相应地，风险评估包括三个部分：危害评估、暴露评估和背景评估。根据上述三个部分的评估结果，描述风险水平（图2）。

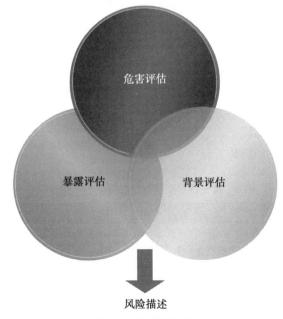

图2　风险评估过程

风险评估并非总依照危害评估、暴露评估、背景评估这一顺序进行,通常同时进行。风险评估过程中,虽然这三个部分的评估工作是分别进行的,但评估所用信息会有部分重叠(见图2)。

危害评估

危害评估是指识别导致事件发生的(一种或一系列)危害及其相关的不良健康后果。公共卫生危害可能是生物性、化学性、物理性及核放射性等危害。危害评估的过程包括:

- 识别可能导致事件发生的危害
- 回顾潜在危害的关键信息(例如:危害特征描述)
- 当存在多个导致事件的危害时,按其发生可能性大小进行排序(等同于临床医学中鉴别诊断)

当事件发生的原因可根据实验室、临床结果或流行病学特征确定时,危害识别相对容易,在此情况下,危害评估通常首先着眼于已知的或高度怀疑的危害。然而多数情况下,危害并不明确,危害评估首先应基于事件的初步描述(例如临床和流行病学特征)、受影响社区的已知疾病负担以及已有危害的类型和分布(例如化工厂及化学物的数量和分布),列出一系列可能的危害。

临床医生、护士、兽医以及其他临床工作者应该十分熟悉的临床鉴别诊断过程,危害评估与之相似。

如果报告的突发公共卫生事件信息越笼统,需列出的可能危害就越多。相反,随着收集到的信息逐渐详尽,潜在的危害数量也随之减少,并且可根据其导致事件发生的可能性排序。

某一事件发生原因的可能性大小取决于:

- 某一疾病在人类或动物中的临床表现及自然史
- 事件发生的时间和进展的速度
- 波及地区和环境
- 涉及的个体和群体特征

表3 某一特定危害可能性评估的问题示例

问题示例
• 可疑危害(病原、毒素、污染物等)能否引起观察到的临床症状和体征?
• 可疑危害是否导致人类或动物患病?
• 涉及的年龄、性别或职业人群是否为危害所累及的典型人群?
• 病例是否有近期旅行史?
• 从可能暴露到出现临床症状的时间是否符合已知特定危害的潜伏期?
• 疾病严重性是否与已知的特定危害或危害类型相同?

续表

问题示例
● 特异的治疗措施（如抗生素）对该疾病是否有效？
● 在往年同期、相同地区或相同人群中，是否曾发生过该可疑危害所导致的疾病？
● 事件发生前是否发生过相关或先兆事件（如动物中疾病暴发或死亡，食物或产品召回，化学性、生物性、核放射性事故或人为释放，邻国发生类似事件等）？
● 实验室检测结果是否确认某一病因或是否与某特定类型的危害一致？

暴露评估

暴露评估是指对个体或群体暴露于可能危害的评估，主要回答以下问题：

- 已暴露或可能暴露于危害的个人或群体数量
- 暴露个体或群体中易感者的数量（例如因未接受免疫接种而可能染病）

进行暴露评估时，需要收集的信息有：

- 传播模式（如通过飞沫或直接接触的人 - 人传播、动物 - 人传播）
- 剂量 - 反应关系（某些特定病原体、毒素或化学性物质）
- 潜伏期（已知或估计）
- 病死率（CFR）
- 传播能力的估计（如 R0，即再生数）
- 暴露人群的免疫接种情况

对于诸如重金属、沙门菌、核辐射等危害，剂量 - 反应关系对于确定暴露强度十分重要；对于此类危害，除了评估暴露本身以外，暴露持续时间同样重要。对于传染病，不同的人群有不同的暴露方式，包括家庭成员（如麻疹）、密切接触者（如 SARS）、社交网络（性传播疾病）、职业暴露人群（乙肝、裂谷热、Q 热）和旅行者（如疟疾）。

对于虫媒疾病（见表 5）和其他动物源性疾病，要进行暴露评估还需收集传播媒介和动物宿主的种类、分布和密度等相关信息。暴露评估可以估计特定地区传播动物源性疾病的可能性。

背景评估

背景评估是指对事件发生的环境所进行的评估，包括对自然环境（如气候、植被、土地使用情况、水源和水利系统）、人群健康状况（如营养状况、疾病负担和既往疫情暴发情况）、基础设施（如交通枢纽、卫生保健、公共卫生设施等）、文化和信仰等各种因素的评估。

具有特定专业领域（如医学、食品安全和兽医）背景的人，在进行风险评估时往往会思路局限于自己熟悉的领域（例如在危害识别过程中），从而忽略其他可能影响风险的因素。

背景评估需要考虑到所有可能的相关因素，概括为 STEEEP[1]，即社会（Social）、科技（Technical）、经济（Economic）、环境（Environmental）、伦理（Ethical）以及政策与政治（Policy&Political）因素（见附录3）。

表4中所列信息可帮助回答以下背景评估中需要解决的关键问题：

● 环境、健康状态、行为、社会和文化背景、基础医疗设施、政策及法律等相关因素中，哪些可能增加人群的脆弱性？

● 环境、健康状态、社会和文化等相关因素中，是否存在可降低人群暴露风险的因素？

● 所有疑似病例均被发现的可能性？

● 有效预防措施、根治或支持性治疗的可用性和可接受程度？

表4 背景评估中可能收集的信息类型示例

信息来源	信息类型	评估产出
监测系统	● 受影响地区运行良好的监测点数量 ● 疑似病例如何被识别	发现病例的可能性
卫生服务基础设施评估或报告	● 受影响地区卫生服务设施的数量、位置和质量 ● 受影响人群的就医行为	病例就医和接受治疗并被治愈的可能性
非政府组织或政府的营养调查报告	● 受影响地区或特定高危人群的营养不良水平	严重疾病发生的可能性
动物和媒介的信息	● 适宜潜在病原媒介大量繁殖的环境信息 ● 潜在动物宿主的数量和分布信息	人群或动物中疾病暴发的可能性

虫媒传染病中的乙脑常被作为危害评估、暴露评估和背景评估中的信息来源示例（见表5）。

表5 乙脑危害评估、暴露评估、背景评估中的信息来源

评估特征		信息来源
危害评估		
病毒因素	基因型别 神经毒性 抗原性 增殖	已发表的关于人类和动物的研究文献 如核苷酸序列数据库（GenBank） 参比实验室数据
临床因素	临床表现 临床进展 严重程度	医学记录（ICD-10）[2]，哨点医院监测系统，实验室监测系统

---

[1] 一些作者将 STEEEP 简写为 PEST 分析，省略其中代表环境 environment 和伦理 ethical 的 E，增加代表环境 environment 和法律 legal 的首字母 E 和 L，缩写为 PESTLE；也有直接添加代表伦理 ethics 的首字母 E，缩写为 STEEPLE。

[2] http://www.who.int/classifications/icd/en/

续表

评估特征		信息来源
暴露评估		
媒介因素	可传播疾病蚊媒的分布、密度和嗜血习性	已发表数据（如昆虫学调查），媒介控制项目数据（如昆虫监测系统包括蚊虫诱捕、乙脑病毒检测方法、杀虫剂敏感性等信息）
宿主因素	人和其他哺乳动物（终末宿主）的感染和疾病的流行病学特征	文献检索，包括血清流行病学研究和暴发调查地方性流行及易于流行地区的指标和事件监测系统（包括人和动物） 病历、基于医院的哨点监测系统，实验室监测系统 全球事件监测系统，包括 Biocaster、GIDEON、GPHIN、HealthMap、EMM MediSys、ProMED Mail、RSOE EDIS 等媒体信息整合系统 流行地区永久性神经损害调查 WHO、FAO、OIE、其他联合国组织、非政府组织（如 PATH）、基金会、慈善机构（如 SciDevNet）、流行国家政府网站等的官方数据和报告。WHO 网站所报告的内容包括疾病暴发新闻（Disease Outbreak News）、流行病学周报（Weekly Epidemiological Record）和需要密码登录的供 IHR 国家归口单位使用的事件信息系统（Event Information Site）及 GOARN 共享平台 可共享的流行病学系统 归国旅行者的病例报告
	扩增宿主（猪和水鸟）的分布和易感性	水鸟数量，与人类密切接触的家猪和野猪的密度与分布情况 猪哨点监测系统数据
	易感性（年龄、人群免疫水平、疫苗覆盖率、交叉抗体的免疫保护情况，如登革热）	病历和病历核查记录（ICD-10[5]、急性神经系统综合征等）
背景评估		
社会经济因素	高危人群数量 农业和牲畜管理	生命统计数据 人口统计数据，包括家庭收入信息（如人口普查）——个人防蚊虫叮咬设备的可及性 人口密度图 流行地区猪养殖业的经济分析
	人类行为	人群对于乙脑病毒传播相关知识知晓情况的调查和研究；预防和控制；关于养猪厂饲养方式；乙脑疫苗接种的可接受性与接种情况等 国际运输（如媒介和生猪）
生态学因素	气候	气象数据（降雨、气温和风力） 气候变化模型数据（如世界气象组织）

续表

评估特征		信息来源
生态学因素	蚊虫孳生地	昆虫学调查；积水分布图；村庄规划，孳生地环境工程控制情况报告 植被覆盖情况的遥感数据，如美国航空航天局（NASA）地球天文台观测系统，全球观测系统信息中心（GOSIC）
	鸟类扩增宿主	鸟的迁徙模式、季节性以及湿地的面积
	野猪	野生动物监测系统；野生动物扑杀项目数据等
项目相关因素	卫生系统能力（急救服务和重症监护服务的可及性、诊断能力、监测系统、乙脑免疫项目、媒介控制项目、经费和人力资源、控制项目的政策支持包括与农业、畜牧业和野生动物机构之间的协作）	全国健康指标数据 常规项目数据、年度报告、项目评估报告等 免疫接种覆盖率数据（已发表的和快速评估，公立和私人医疗机构相关数据等）

风险描述

在风险评估团队完成对危害、暴露和背景的评估后，依据评估结果可确定风险水平，此过程为风险描述。风险描述可以依据定量模型或通过与已有标准进行对比（例如食品安全风险评估）计算出相应数值；当缺乏具体数值时，风险水平的判断则基于专家团队的意见。

风险矩阵是风险描述的有效辅助工具（见图 3a 和图 3b），可用于整合危害发生可能性（见表 6）及其发生后果的严重性（见表 7）。

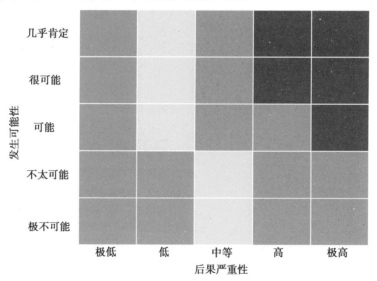

图 3a　分类边界明确的风险矩阵

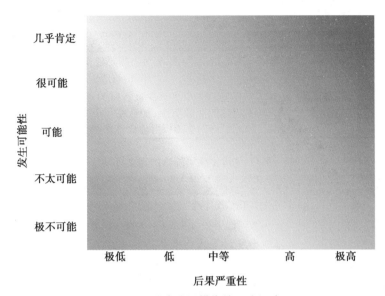

图 3b　分类边界模糊的风险矩阵

　　鉴于大多数突发公共卫生事件的风险评估是定性评估,因此在风险矩阵中的分类并非基于数值而是基于发生可能性和后果严重性宽泛的定性描述(表6、表7和图3a、图3b的图例对如何理解风险矩阵进行解释)。

　　当使用风险矩阵时,发生可能性和后果严重性的定义应与该国或该地区的背景相适应。

　　图3a和图3b展示了两种风险矩阵,评估团队可依据需求选择矩阵类型;两种矩阵均为直观可视化工具,可以激发进一步的讨论并帮助确定风险水平。

　　讨论过程中,评估团队不仅仅要考虑预期发病率、死亡率以及与事件直接相关的长期健康损害(如残疾),而且应考虑其所有后果。附表3提供了需考虑的 STEEEP 后果。

　　风险矩阵还可以用于评价和记录采取控制措施前后风险的变化。在评估某些事件时,如可用信息十分有限或风险水平非常明确,则可能不需使用风险矩阵。

表 6　如何解读图 3a 和图 3b[1]

	风险水平	采取的行动
	低风险	根据标准响应方案、常规控制项目和规范进行管理(如通过常规监测系统进行跟踪)
	中等风险	明确响应的职责和分工,需要采取特定的监测和控制措施(如加强监测,强化免疫)

[1]　改编自 WHO 和 FAO. *Risk Characterization of Microbiological Hazards in Food*. Microbiological Risk Assessment Series 17, World Health Organization and Food and Agriculture Organization, 1999.(http://www.who.int/foodsafety/publications/micro/MRA17.pdf).

续表

风险水平	采取的行动
高风险	需要高级别的应急响应:可能需要建立应急指挥和控制架构;需要采取一系列应急控制措施,某些措施会产生显著的影响
极高风险	需要立即响应,即使事件报告时为非正常工作时间。立即启动高级别的应急响应(如应在几小时内建立指挥和控制架构);控制措施的实施极可能会带来严重的影响

表7　风险发生可能性的定义 [1]

等级	定义
几乎肯定	绝大多数情况下会发生(如发生概率≥95%)
很可能	大多数情况下很可能发生(如发生概率70%～94%)
可能	有时会发生(如发生概率30%～69%)
不太可能	有时可能会发生(如发生概率5%～29%)
极不可能	极个别情况下发生(如发生概率<5%)

表8　风险发生后果的定义 [1]

等级	后果
极低	对所涉及人群的影响有限 对正常生产、生活几乎没有影响 常规响应足以应对,无需采取应急控制措施 政府和利益相关者需投入的附加费用极少
低	对少部分人群或高危人群有轻微的影响 对正常生产、生活的影响有限 需要采取少量的应急控制措施,需要消耗少量资源 政府和利益相关者需投入少量附加费用
中等	对较多的人群或高危人群产生一定程度的影响 对正常生产、生活产生一定程度的破坏 需要一些应急控制措施,需消耗一定量的资源 政府和利益相关者需投入一定量的附加费用
高	对少部分人群或高危人群产生严重影响 对正常生产、生活造成严重的破坏 需强有力的应急控制措施,需消耗大量资源 政府和利益相关者需投入的附加费用明显增加
极高	对大规模人群或高危人群产生极严重的影响 对正常生产、生活造成极严重的破坏 需强有力的应急控制措施,需消耗大量资源 政府和利益相关者需投入的附加费用急剧增加

---

[1] 改编自 WHO 和 FAO. *Risk Characterization of Microbiological Hazards in Food*. Microbiological Risk Assessment Series 17, World Health Organization and Food and Agriculture Organization, 1999.(http://www.who.int/foodsafety/publications/micro/MRA17.pdf).

风险评估的可信度

风险评估团队对本次风险评估的可信度与局限性分析记录十分重要[1]。风险评估的可信度取决于评估所用信息的可靠性及完整性，以及基于危害、暴露、背景资料做出的基本假设。

关于危害、暴露和背景的信息和证据越多，风险评估结果的可信度越高。可信度可以用描述性分级来表述（极低到极高）。

表9展示了确定风险评估结果可信度的两种情形。示例A描述了来自各种来源的详细信息，包括临床一手资料、当地信息、历史记录、经过同行评议的文章；基于这些信息的风险评估可信度可达到中等或高水平。与之相比，示例B的事件来自报纸文章报道，未被其他渠道确认；单独依据该信息所进行的风险评估可信度为低或极低。

表9　两个风险评估的可信度

示例A：可信度高	示例B：可信度低
危害评估基于以下资料： ● 临床医生提供的病例详细临床信息 ● 过去两年该病原造成类似暴发事件 ● 监测数据	危害评估基于以下资料： ● 报纸文章所报道的非专业的病例信息 ● 报告中未提及历史数据
暴露评估基于以下资料： ● 快速应急队伍的流行病学调查 ● 同行评议文章和来自既往暴发的证据	暴露评估基于以下资料： ● 基于媒体报道的临床特征所推测的可能传播途径（如表现为恶心、呕吐、腹泻的急性传染病可能经食物或水传播）
背景评估基于以下资料： ● 既往暴发期间卫生服务系统的运转情况 ● 外部评议 ● 来自当地官方或卫生部门的详细信息	背景评估基于以下资料： ● 风险评估团队中某个工作人员的知识和经验

框2　风险描述示例——严重呼吸系统疾病

事件概况：过去17天内，X国家共报告聚集性严重呼吸系统疾病病例22例、死亡7人。事件由一地方医务工作者（HCW）报告，事发地距离边境8公里，病例分布于三个村庄。该地区是X国内的贫困地区，医疗设施简陋。由于当地许多卫生保健机构向病人收取就诊费，所以当地人病情轻微时常常自行服药。当地认为该次怪病由巫术所致。

风险问题：该严重呼吸系统疾病是否存在进一步扩散的可能？扩散后的公共卫生影响（包括影响的类型和程度）如何？

用于评估疫情进一步扩散可能性的信息：

● 首例病例发现17天后仍然有病例报告；

---

[1] 有些情况下，在评估时不用"可信度"或"确定性"，而用其反义词"不确定性"（参见附录2）。

- 具体的危害和传播模式尚不明确；
- 部分病例可能尚未被发现（如轻症病例很可能未就医而未纳入官方病例统计）

因此，如不及时采取行动，很可能还会有病例发生。

用于评估疫情进一步扩散导致后果的信息：

- 该疾病具有高病死率（即使将部分未报告病例考虑在内）；
- 当地卫生服务系统能力和对病例救治的能力较弱；新增病例会给急诊医疗服务带来较大负担，致使住院病例临床转归更加不容乐观；
- 病例和死亡对受影响社区带来不良的经济和社会影响；
- 当地人深信是巫术导致的死亡，可能带来社会的不安定；
- 该事件发生于边境地区，可能存在跨境传播的风险。

因此，如果病例进一步增加，该事件的后果将为严重。

使用风险矩阵综合考虑事件发生的可能性和后果的严重性，进而得出该事件的总体风险水平为高。

本次风险评估的可信度为低 - 中等。

尽管报告信息来自一名地方医务工作者，但信息量有限，尚不清楚该医务工作者是否诊治过疑似病例，还是仅根据传闻来报告。

通常在开展一系列风险评估的起始阶段，风险评估结果的可信度都不高（参见表9中的示例B），评估结果依赖于专家团队的意见以及对有限信息的解读。

需要强调的是，可信度低的风险评估并不代表是低质量的风险评估，相反，评估结果反映了进行评估时可用的信息有限。因此，对风险评估得出的每一个结论和建议作出可信度评估十分重要（见框2）。

定量风险评估

风险评估中的定量程度受多重因素影响，如评估资料的可用性、评估时限要求、评估问题的复杂程度等。

在诸如工程学等领域中，精确定量的风险评估是可行的；但是在突发公共卫生事件的风险评估中，尤其是事件发生初期资料比较匮乏时，定性风险评估可能是唯一选择。

尽管某些生物学风险评估历时多年（如在国际贸易领域中，由多学科组成的评估团队耗时数年完成），但也很难保证在评估的各个步骤都可以应用可信的定量指标进行评估。在实际工作中，多数风险评估都是采用定性和定量相结合的方法进行。当可获得定量信息时就采用定量评估，不可获得时就采用定性评估。

需要注意的是，用质量差的数据或错误的方法所进行的定量风险评估所得出的结果，远不及一个设计良好的定性风险评估的结果科学可信。附录4提供了关于风险评估中定量研究的详细信息。

控 制 措 施

　　应当根据风险评估的结果采取恰当的控制措施,确认总体风险水平有助于确定所需采取控制措施的紧迫性和强度。

　　也可以用类似风险矩阵的方法根据防控效果对控制措施进行分级。例如,可列出每一种控制措施防止危害进一步扩散或传播的可能性等级(见表10),及其实施导致不良后果的等级(见表11)。

表10　控制措施的有效性

等级	定义
肯定有效	在多数情况下,能够防止新病例的发生
很可能有效	在多数情况下,很可能防止新病例的发生
可能有效	在某些情况下,能够防止新病例的发生
不太有效	在某些情况下,可能防止新病例的发生
基本无效	在特殊情况下,可能防止新病例的发生

表11　控制措施实施的不良后果

等级	定义
极低	社会影响:有限
	伦理问题:无
	经济影响:无或轻微
	政治影响:无或轻微
低	社会影响:低
	伦理问题:有限
	经济影响:有限
	政治影响:有些
中等	社会影响:中等
	伦理问题:有些
	经济影响:中等
	政治影响:中等

续表

等级	定义
高	社会影响：高
	伦理问题：显著
	经济影响：高
	政治影响：高
极高	社会影响：极高
	伦理问题：大量
	经济影响：极高
	政治影响：极高

　　风险评估小组应该考虑附录 3 中各项控制措施的 STEEEP 后果，因此，应囊括 STEEEP 中列出的所有因素，而不是仅考虑部分后果（例如，评估时只考虑控制措施对科学技术或生物医药方面的影响）。

　　评估控制措施的有效性与后果有助于判断该措施对于控制某种危害风险是否恰当，帮助评估小组说服决策者采取最适当控制措施，或协助决策者确定可接受风险水平。

　　一般情况下，控制效果为"肯定有效"且不良影响为"低～中等"水平的控制措施最易被接受。但在某些特殊情况下，例如，高风险（即几乎肯定将导致严重的后果）和（或）可信度低的事件需要采取谨慎的或预防性策略，那些控制效果即使仅为"可能有效"的控制措施也可接受。

风 险 沟 通

风险沟通是风险管理过程中不可分割的一部分,详见附录5。它包含两个同等重要的部分:

● 业务沟通:机构为了达到工作目的和战略目标而采用的结构化沟通方式,包括协调机构内外的成员和团体。它在风险评估组与利益相关者(技术专家和相应政府层级的决策者、其他响应机构或私营机构等)之间进行;

● 公众沟通:是指定期将风险评估的主要结论告知公众。它可以确保公众了解风险的性质和严重程度以及可采取的最有效的预防控制措施。

开展风险评估时,评估小组应首先确定利益相关者,并尽快制定沟通策略以确保风险管理组与利益相关者间的双向沟通。

沟通策略应包含:

● 风险评估小组以何种形式将风险评估进行定期反馈;

● 明确风险沟通中的角色和职责(如联络点);

● 以何种形式将相关信息传递给利益相关者及公众。

监督与评价

风险评估应随着信息的更新而再次开展，也可以定期开展（例如，在一起事件初期，每天开展风险评估也许是因为某位部长同意每天同一时间向其他部长或者媒体通报事件进展）。

每次风险评估都应基于该事件上次的评估结论。每次风险评估都应记录在案（包括评估时使用数据和信息），这些记录对于监督和评价风险评估过程是不可或缺的资料。

由于事件的规模和复杂性，随着公共卫生事件的进展风险评估可能需要解决新的和不同的风险问题。对于某些事件，可能需要不同风险评估小组的协作以掌握事件风险的全貌（例如，临床症状严重程度、传播动力学和控制措施）。

对事件进行总结时，应正式回顾所有风险评估结果。系统分析良好记录的风险评估可以发现突发公共卫生事件管理中需要改进之处。

附录1：本手册名词术语

可接受风险 Acceptable risk	可以容忍或可以接受的风险水平。应对危害进行监控以识别可能导致风险增加的任何改变。确定可接受风险水平时需要考虑利益相关者的知情同意，并且应考虑"可接受性"在不同利益相关者、人群、地域以及文化中会有明显不同。
突发公共卫生事件 Acute public health event	任何可能对人类健康造成负面影响的事件。包括尚未引起人类疾病，但可能会通过受污染/感染的食物、水、动物、产品或环境而引起人类疾病的事件。
突发事件公共卫生风险 Acute pubic health risk	突发事件对公众健康造成负面影响的风险。
预警 Alert	对已经发生或即将发生的可能导致不良后果的公共卫生事件所进行的首次通告。
全危害策略 All-hazards approach	在突发事件管理中，将所有潜在危害纳入分析评估的策略。包括生物性、化学性、放射性危害以及自然灾害（如火灾、水灾、其他极端天气情况、火山爆发、地震及海啸）。
偏倚 Bias	导致研究结果或推论与真实情况产生差异的系统误差。
可信度 Confidence	评估组对其评估结论的把握度。它相当于某些领域评估中使用的确定性或不确定性。即使掌握的信息近乎完美（即不存在不确定信息），自然存在的变异还会使评估存在不确定性。
确认 Confirmation	通过收集证据核实信息的准确性并得出结论的过程（例如，信息已经过认证）。
后果 Consequences	某种行动或条件造成的下游影响，影响可能是正面或负面的。负面的公共卫生后果导致人群健康水平降低。影响可能包括社会、技术、科学、经济、环境、伦理、政策以及政治等多方面。
背景评估 Context assessment	对事件发生所处环境进行的评估。
控制措施 Control measures	为减轻危害对暴露人群的影响所采取的干预措施。
发现 Detection	采用系统的方法发觉突发事件。

鉴别诊断 Differential Diagnosis	通过分析患者的健康相关数据及性别、年龄等其他关键信息而做出诊断的系统方法。
事件监测 Event-based Surveillance	有组织地快速收集具有潜在公共卫生风险的事件信息。
事件报告 Event report	系统记录某事件的时间、人群、地区（包括背景）相关信息的报告。
暴露评估 Exposure assessment	针对已确认的危害，评价个人或群体的潜在暴露。
假阳性 False positive	实际无病，但被某检验结果判断为有病。
危害 Hazard	可能造成暴露人群健康损害的因子。
危害评估 Hazard assessment	识别可能导致事件发生的危害及其可能引起的不良健康影响。
IHR	国际卫生条例（2005）。
IHR 联络点 IHR Contact Point	与国际卫生条例缔约国归口单位沟通联系的世界卫生组织联络点。
IHR 国家归口单位 IHR National Focal Point	根据国际卫生条例，缔约国指定的可与 WHO 及其成员国随时进行联络的部门或机构。
IHR 报告 IHR Report	缔约国收发《国际卫生条例》规定的可能引起国际关注的突发公共卫生事件的报告。
指标监测 Indicator-based Surveillance	根据病例定义 [1] 以及预先设定的指标常规收集信息（例如弛缓性麻痹病例的每周监测）。通常预先设定有预警和响应的暴发阈值。
传染病 Infectious disease	传染性病原或其产生的毒素，由感染病例、动物或储存宿主传播给易感宿主所导致的疾病。
可能性 Likelihood	事件发生的概率。
NGO	非政府组织。
暴发 Outbreak	表现为局部地区发病率升高的疾病流行。
公共卫生 Public health	为了促进人群健康而计划并实施的健康项目及服务，包括认识并降低发病、残疾和死亡的风险。

---

[1] 该处"疾病"为广义，包括综合征。

预防性措施 Precautionary approach	1992 年联合国环境与发展大会上发表的里约声明第 15 条原则首次在全球层面对"预防性措施"进行了界定。该原则指出,即使缺乏科学证据,也不能推迟为避免对环境产生严重或不可逆转的损害而采取的行动。该原则在多个领域均适用,包括公共卫生领域。注意:该原则可能并不适用于其他领域(如在输入性风险评估中,采取的行动应谨慎或保守,而不提倡"预防性措施"原则)。
可靠性 Reliability	在相同条件下,用某测量工具重复测量同一受试对象获得相同结果的稳定程度。
风险 Risk	在特定时期内,发生不良事件的可能性及其后果的严重程度。
风险评估 Risk assessment	通过收集、评价、记录信息,确定风险等级的系统过程。包括三个环节:危害评估、暴露评估和背景评估。
风险沟通 Risk communication	风险沟通是为了进行依据充分的决策、使目标人群做出积极的行为改变以及维持相关机构或个人间的相互信任,贯穿于公共卫生事件的准备期、应对期以及恢复期,在责任机构、合作机构以及受威胁社区间的一系列沟通原则、活动以及信息交换的统称。
风险管理 Risk management	依据风险评估的结果权衡可选择的政策的过程,必要时进一步选择并采取恰当的干预措施。对于突发公共卫生事件,风险管理是选择并采取恰当的措施以达到控制和减轻突发公共卫生风险不良后果的过程。
风险描述 Risk statement	对确定的突发公共卫生事件风险等级进行的描述,该描述应包含对所确定的风险等级的可信度。
灵敏度 Sensitivity	实际阳性者按某检验标准被正确判断为阳性的比例。如:实际有病而按某检验标准被正确判断为有病的百分比。
综合征 Syndrome	一组总是同时出现的临床体征和症状,或以一系列相关的临床体征和症状为特征的疾病状态。
筛选 Triage	判断经监测系统发现的事件或预警是否对公众健康有潜在风险以及是否优先对其做出响应的过程。
脆弱性 Vulnerability	相对不利的状态。个体或群体无法预防或应对危害的程度。
动物源性疾病 Zoonosis (plural: zoonoses)	能在人和动物间传播的疾病。

附录2：不同部门和学科使用的定义

食品安全风险分析所用术语

食品法典委员会（Codex）规定食品风险分析的三个组成部分：
- 风险评估
- 风险管理
- 风险沟通

法典规定的食品安全风险分析方法的三个步骤：

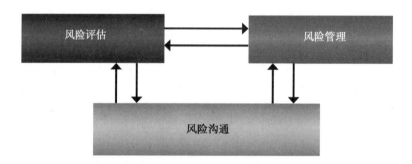

食品安全风险分析中，使用的术语定义如下：

- 危害：食品中所含有的可能引起不良健康影响的生物性、化学性或物理性因子或状况。

- 风险：是描述食品中危害造成的不良健康影响的可能性及影响的严重程度。

- 风险分析：该过程包括三个部分：风险评估，风险管理和风险沟通。

- 风险评估：是一个基于科学的过程，包括以下几个步骤，1.危害识别；2.危害特征描述；3.暴露评估；4.风险特征描述。

- 危害识别：识别某特定食品或某类食品中能够导致不良健康影响的生物性、化学性和物理性因子。

- 危害特征描述：对食品中的生物、化学或物理性因子引起的不良健康影响的性质进行定性或定量评估的过程。对于化学性因子，应该进行剂量 - 反应评估；对于生物性或物理性因子，如果可以获得数据，也应当进行剂量 - 反应评估。

● 暴露评估：对通过食物或其他相关来源摄入的生物性、化学性、物理性因子的摄入量进行定量和（或）定性评估的过程。

● 风险特征描述：在危害识别、危害特征描述和暴露评估的基础上，定性和（或）定量地估计特定人群在特定暴露状态下出现不良反应的可能性及严重程度，包括不确定性描述。

● 风险管理：与风险评估不同，风险管理是为了保护消费者健康、促进公平贸易，选择适宜的预防和控制措施，通过与所有利益相关方协商，并综合考虑风险评估结果及其他相关因素、以权衡选择政策的过程。

● 风险沟通：在风险分析全过程中，风险评估者、风险管理者、消费者、企业、学术机构以及其他利益相关方就危害、风险、风险相关因素以及风险认知方面交换信息和观点的过程，包括解释风险评估结果和风险管理决策的基本原理。

输入风险分析所用术语

世界动物卫生组织（OIE）制定的陆生及水生动物卫生法典（Codes）中描述了输入风险分析的 4 个部分：

● 危害识别

● 风险评估

● 风险管理

● 风险沟通

世界动物卫生组织制定的输入风险分析 4 个部分：

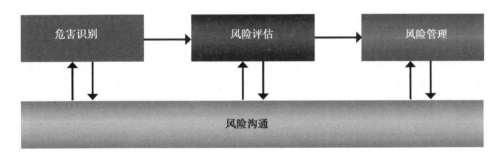

输入风险分析中，世界动物卫生组织使用的术语定义如下：

● 危害：任何可能对商品输入造成不良后果的病原体。

● 风险：在特定时期内，会对输入国的动物和人群造成危害的不良事件的发生可能性及其影响程度。

● 风险分析：危害识别、风险评估、风险管理和风险沟通的过程。

● 危害识别：识别可能随商品而输入的病原体的过程。

● 风险评估：评估病原体在输入国定殖并传播的可能性及其造成的生物和经济后果。

● 风险管理：明确、选择并执行某种可降低风险水平措施的过程。

● 风险沟通：风险评估者、风险管理者和其他利益相关团体交流风险信息的过程。

扩展阅读：

Anderson K et al., eds. The Economics of Quarantine and the SPS Agreement. Centre for International Economic Studies, Adelaide, and AFFA Biosecurity Australia, Canberra, 2001.

Aven T. Foundations of Risk Analysis: a knowledge and decision-oriented perspective. John Wiley andSons, Chichester, 2003.

Byrd DM and Cothern RC Introduction to Risk Analysis: A systematic approach to science-based decision making. Government Institutes, Rockville, Maryland, 2000.

Codex. Risk Assessment Procedures used by the Codex Alimentarius Commission and its Subsidiary and Advisory Bodies. Codex Alimentarius Commission, Food and Agriculture Organization, Geneva, 1993.

Covello VT and Merkhofer MW. Risk Assessment Methods: approaches for assessing health and environmental risks, Plenum Press, New York, 1993.

Flynn J et al., eds. Risk, Media and Stigma: understanding public challenges to modern science and technology. Earthscan.London, 2001.

Morgan MG and Henrion M. Uncertainty: a guide to dealing with uncertainty in quantitative risk and policy analysis. Cambridge University Press, Cambridge, 1992.

OIE.Handbook on Import Risk Analysis for Animals and Animal Products. 2nd ed: Introduction and qualitative risk analysis. World Organisation for Animal Health, Paris, 2010.

OIE.Handbook on Import Risk Analysis for Animals and Animal Products. 2nd ed: Quantitative risk analysis. World Organisation for Animal Health, Paris, 2010.

OIE. Aquatic Animal Health Code(published online at http: //www.oie.int/international-standardsetting/aquatic-code/access-online/). World Organisation for Animal Health, Paris, 2011.

OIE.Terrestrial Animal Health Code.(published online at http://www.oie.int/international-standardsetting/terrestrial-code/access-online/). World Organisation for Animal Health, Paris, 2011.

Renn O, ed. Risk Governance: coping with uncertainty in a complex world. Earthscan. London, 2008.

Robertson D and Kellow A, eds. Globalization and the Environment: risk assessment and the WTO. Edward Elgar, Cheltenham, United Kingdom, 2001.

Vose DJ. Quantitative Risk Analysis: a guide to Monte Carlo modelling, 2nd ed. John Wiley and Sons, Chichester, 2000.

附录3：突发公共事件及其控制措施的 STEEEP 后果示例

社会（Social）

- 对被隔离个体的影响，特别是当隔离医院远离其居住社区时
- 限制接触的影响（例如，限制家人探视感染者或重症患者）
- 重要社交或宗教活动的改变（例如，社交距离政策）
- 对生活方式的影响（例如，儿童看护方式的改变）
- 受影响的社区对干预措施的接受程度
- 传染病患者受到的歧视
- 心理影响

技术与科学（Technical and scientific）

- 发病率、死亡率和长期伤残率
- 控制措施的有效性
- 及时采取控制措施的能力
- 治疗和预防的副作用

经济（Economic）

- 应急准备与响应机构的直接经济费用
- 受影响的个人、家庭、社区采取措施的直接经济费用（例如，医疗费、护理费、畜养牲畜损失）
- 间接损失：
- ——对个人或家庭工作的影响（例如，学校关闭、家庭隔离、住院）
- ——对家庭收入的影响
- ——对社区收入的影响
- ——对国民经济的影响
- 从当地、国家和全球层面考虑以下方面：
- ——对旅行和贸易的影响
- ——对旅游业的影响

环境（Environmental）

- 控制措施对自然环境的负面影响（例如，污染或残留）
- 对自然环境的正面影响（例如，通过控制虫媒同时控制了其他可能发生的疾病）

伦理（Ethical）

- 个人自由（比如限制活动）
- 非预期的结果（当家禽被捕杀，污染的粮食被销毁，又没有其他可供选择的食物时，家庭失去了最主要的食物来源）

续表

- 个人隐私
- 保护公众免受伤害
- 使用未经有关部门许可的药品或疫苗
- 知情同意(人们理解他们被要求接受或允许的事项)
- 使社区群体和个人免受歧视(例如,被认为是没有价值的或者得不到赞同)
- 适宜性(控制措施与风险水平相适应)
- 提供关怀的责任(例如,有义务向个人或人群提供安全、专业和符合伦理的关怀)
- 平等(公平无偏见)
- 透明(例如,公开、明显、明白)
- 不平等的风险负担(例如,医护人员,其他一线应对工作者)

政策与政治(Policy and political)

- 应急响应机构高层管理者的观点(例如,与其他项目或政策的相容性)[1]
- 为了支持应对工作需要从其他项目或计划中进行的资源分流
- 卫生部部长及其他部长的观点
- 反对团体的观点
- 即将到来的大选或其他重要政治事件
- 媒体和主要利益相关团体可能做出的反应
- 政府无意愿或无能力进行有效应对(例如,政治迫害或武装冲突;为国内转移安置者或难民提供可及医疗保健服务)

---

[1] 有时被称为项目风险。

附录4: 定量风险评估

风险评估的量化水平取决于可利用的信息、所要求的评估速度和问题的复杂性等因素。

一些文献指出存在两种风险评估的方法:定性(不用或只用少量的数据)和定量(运用数据和计算机建模)。然而,即使最纯粹的定量方法也都依赖于定性的、主观的判断来建立模型及估计参数。同样,最纯粹的定性方法也涉及对风险、后果进行排序,因此其包含了定量的性质,因为排序即是数理概率论和形式逻辑的体现。

结构化正规风险评估可以使用多种不同的方法,包括基于生物系统描述的主观推理、点得分系统、逻辑规则以及蒙特卡罗模拟。风险评估还可用不同的数量水平,即不同程度的定量化表达评估信息和分析结果。

在一些学科中,例如工程学,高度定量化的风险评估被广泛应用。即使在持续两年或更长时间的生物风险评估中(例如,在国际贸易中,庞大的多学科团队合作进行重要输入风险评估),并非每个评估阶段都可以获得可靠的定量数据资料。实践中,许多评估综合运用多种方法,数据多时使用定量方法,数据少时则使用定性方法。突发公共卫生事件风险评估中,特别在事件早期可得的数据有限时,定性方法可能是唯一选择。

可使用敏感性分析确定某不易得到的特定参数对整体风险估计的影响。这类敏感性分析常常显示,一种方法(一个过程)中仅有少数的关键点对整体的风险有较大影响。如果可以获得这些关键点上的相关数据,则风险评估会更加可信和稳健。然而,如果无法获得这些关键点的理想数据,风险评估中就应该尽量避免运用定量的方法,除非通过实施恰当的研究获取所需的数据。

定量方法并非一定优于定性方法。如果定量风险评估中使用了低质量的数据或不恰当的技术,则其科学性和可靠性都远差于定性研究。构架良好、及时的定性评估优于不完整的、滞后的定量评估。

贸易方面,符合世界贸易组织(WTO)关于卫生和植物检疫措施应用协定(SPS协定)的所有定量评估都是可接受的。WTO承认与环境相适应的纯定性研究也是有效的。

扩展阅读：

Anderson K et al., eds. The Economics of Quarantine and the SPS Agreement. Centre for International Economic Studies, Adelaide, and AFFA Biosecurity Australia, Canberra, 2001.

Aven T. Foundations of Risk Analysis: a knowledge and decision-oriented perspective. John Wiley and Sons, Chichester, 2003.

Byrd DM and Cothern, RC. Introduction to Risk Analysis: A systematic approach to science-based decision making. Government Institutes, Rockville, Maryland, 2000.

Codex. Risk Assessment Procedures used by the Codex Alimentarius Commission and its Subsidiary and Advisory Bodies. Codex Alimentarius Commission, Food and Agriculture Organization, Geneva, 1993.

Covello, VT and Merkhofer MW. Risk Assessment Methods: Approaches for assessing health and environmental risks, Plenum Press, New York, 1993.

Morgan MG and Henrion M. Uncertainty: a guide to dealing with uncertainty in quantitative risk and policy analysis. Cambridge University Press, Cambridge, 1992.

OIE. International Aquatic Animal Health Code (published online at: http://www.oie.int/eng/normes/fcode/A_summry.htm). World Organisation for Animal Health, Paris, 2003.

OIE. Terrestrial Animal Health Code (published online at: http://www.oie.int/eng/normes/mcode/A_summry.htm). World Organisation for Animal Health, Paris, 2003.

OIE. Handbook on Import Risk Analysis for Animals and Animal Products, 2nd ed. Volume 1: Introduction and qualitative risk analysis. World Organisation for Animal Health, Paris, 2010.

OIE.Handbook on Import Risk Analysis for Animals and Animal Products. Volume 2: Quantitative risk analysis. World Organisation for Animal Health, Paris, 2004.

Robertson D and Kellow A, eds. Globalization and the Environment: risk assessment and the WTO. Edward Elgar, Cheltenham, United Kingdom, 2001.

Vose DJ. Quantitative Risk Analysis: a guide to Monte Carlo modelling, 2nd ed. John Wiley and Sons, Chichester, 2000.

附录5：风险沟通

　　风险沟通是为了进行依据充分的决策，使目标人群做出积极的行为改变以及维持相关机构或个人间的相互信任，贯穿于公共卫生事件的准备期、应对期以及恢复期，在责任机构、合作机构以及受威胁社区间的一系列沟通原则、活动以及信息交换的统称。

　　在风险管理的各个环节中，虽然风险沟通往往被列在最后，这并未正确反映风险沟通的重要性。为了更好发挥风险评估的作用，在风险评估的早期就应制定好风险沟通计划并在评估的每一阶段做好该项工作。否则，风险评估易被理解为专业风险评估者告知利益相关者评估结果，并建议实施他们推荐的管理策略的过程。这种自上而下的方法意味着风险沟通很大程度上是单向的，忽略了在评估整个过程中必要的协商讨论。不良的风险沟通会激发利益相关者的愤怒情绪。

　　由于专家与公众的立场和专业背景不同，风险沟通中经常存在问题。这些情形体现在：专家更多使用专业词汇、统计数据，而公众则更多的使用通俗语言。以下列举出了两种表达方式的区别（改编自 Powell and Leiss，1997）[1]。

专家和公众风险评估

"专家"评估风险	"公众"评估风险
基于科学	靠直觉
关注"可接受风险"	关注安全（无风险）
根据最新信息改变风险认识	风险认识固化
比较不同事件的风险	关注单独的事件风险
关注群体平均水平	关注个体后果
"1 例死亡就是 1 例死亡"	"这关乎到我们的死活"

　　理想的风险沟通是能够用不同语言表达方式融会贯通，使得不同群体都能正确理解沟通的内容。

风险认知

　　利益相关者和公众对风险的认知往往与专业评估者不同。多种因素决定了

---

[1] Powell D and Leiss W. *Mad Cows and Mother's Milk: the perils of poor risk communication*. McGill–Queen's University Press，Montreal，1997.

个体和群体对风险的认知。例如，分析显示，与经统计学证实存在的危害相比，人们通常认为不常见的或引起恐慌的危害会导致更高的风险。人们通常更加重视可能导致灾难性后果的低概率危害，公众会更加强烈要求政府出台相应政策和保护措施。例如核事故，不明原因的动物源性疾病（埃博拉或尼帕病毒），可能导致本地物种大量死亡的已知疾病。风险评估者在与利益相关者交流时需要考虑这些情形，并理解激发群体产生不良情绪的原因。

即使获得了有关危害的重要信息，人们对信息来源的信任程度也会影响对风险的认知。例如，调查显示，与政府（和专家）发布的信息相比，公众更加信任环保团体和消费者组织发布的信息。同样，人们更倾向于相信媒体信息而非政府官方声明。

理想风险沟通的经验

目前已有一些不良风险沟通的案例，例如牛海绵状脑病（BSE 或疯牛病）流行的风险沟通。高技术性行业的风险评估人员常常专注于技术细节。他们可能会惊讶地发现，他们专注从事的风险评估工作和谨慎推理得出的建议竟然会遭到公众强烈的反对。如果不能及时并全程与利益相关者和公众进行风险沟通，而是在风险评估过程的后期才考虑到风险沟通，就很可能会引起公众负面反应。

在对动物健康、食品安全和公共卫生事件案例进行分析研究的基础上，Powell 和 Leis（1997）提出了风险沟通的 10 条经验：

- 事件信息的缺失是风险被社会放大的首要因素
- 管理者应负责开展有效的风险沟通
- 相关行业对有效地开展风险沟通负有责任
- 负责人员要及早并经常开展风险沟通
- "科学"能够解释的风险问题是有限的
- 要始终将科学置于大的政策环境中考虑
- "教育大众"并不能代替理想的风险沟通实践
- 摒弃"无风险"的信息
- 风险信息应该直接回答"有争议的问题"
- 有效的沟通有利于风险管理

附录6：本手册编者

Dr BenidoImpouma, Technical Officer, Epidemic and Pandemic Alert and Response Disease Prevention and Control Cluster, Regional Office for Africa, B.P.6, Brazzaville Republic of Congo

Dr Roberta Andraghetti, Advisor, International Health Regulations, Regional Office for the Americas, Pan American Sanitary Bureau, 525, 23rd Street, N.W. Washington, DC20037, United States of America

Dr Richard Brown, Regional Advisor, Department of Disease Surveillance and Epidemiology, WorldHealth Organization, Regional Office for South-East Asia

Dr Graham Tallis, Medical Officer, Communicable Diseases Surveillance and Response ProgramManager, World Health Organization, Country Office Indonesia

Dr Jukka Tapani Pukkila, Programme Manager, Alert and Response Operations, Division of Communicable Diseases, Health Security, & Environment, World Health Organization, Regional Office for Europe, 8, Scherfigsvej, DK-2100 Copenhagen, Denmark

Dr Shahin Huseynov, Technical Officer, World Health Organization, Country Office Uzbekistan

Dr Langoya Martin Opoka, Technical Officer, Disease Surveillance, Forecasting and Response, World Health Organization, Regional Office for the Eastern Mediterranean, Abdul Razzak Al Sanhouri Street, Nasr City, Cairo 1371, Egypt

Dr Ruth Foxwell, Epidemiologist, Emerging Disease Surveillance and Response, Division of HealthSecurity and Emergencies, World Health Organization, Western Pacific Regional Office, 1000 Manila, Philippines

Dr FrancetteDusan, Veterinary Epidemiologist, formally Communicable Disease Surveillance andResponse, World Health Organisation, Lao PDR

Dr Mike J Nunn, Principal Scientist(Animal Biosecurity), Australian Government Department of Agriculture, Fisheries and Forestry, GPO Box 858, Canberra ACT 2601, Australia

Dr Angela Merianos, Project Leader, Risk Assessment and Decision Support, Alert and Response Operations, Department of Global Alert and Response, World Health Organization, Geneva, Switzerland

Amy Cawthorne, Epidemiologist, Risk Assessment and Decision Support, Alert and Response Operations/ Department of Global Alert and Response, World Health Organization, Geneva, Switzerland

Erika Garcia, Technical Officer, Risk Assessment and Decision Support, Alert and

Response Operations, Department of Global Alert and Response, World Health Organization, Geneva, Switzerland

Dr Stephanie Williams, Medical Officer, formally Risk Assessment and Decision Support, Alert andResponse Operations, Department of Global Alert and Response, World Health Organization, Geneva, Switzerland

Dr Andrea Ellis, Scientist, formally Risk Assessment and Management, Food Safety, Zoonoses and Foodborne Diseases, World Health Organization, Geneva, Switzerland

Dr KerstenGutschmidt, Technical Officer, Evidence and Policy on Emerging EH Issues, World Health Organization, Geneva, Switzerland

Dr Danilo Lo Fo Wong, Coordinator, Antimicrobial Resistance, World Health Organization, Regional Office for Europe, 8, Scherfigsvej, DK-2100 Copenhagen, Denmark

Table of contents

Introduction to the manual

This manual has been developed to guide rapid risk assessment of acute public health risks from any type of hazard in response to requests from Member States of the World Health Organization (WHO). The manual is aimed primarily at national departments with health-protection responsibilities, National Focal Points (NFPs) for the International Heath Regulations (IHR) and WHO staff. It should also be useful to others who join multidisciplinary risk assessment teams, such as clinicians, field epidemiologists, veterinarians, chemists, food-safety specialists.

The manual will assist rapid and defensible decision-making about acute public health events that pose a risk to human health through application of a systematic process from event detection and risk assessment to communication with key stakeholders and the public.

The manual complements existing hazard-specific risk assessment guidance (see Appendices 1 and 2), including:

- *WHO Human Health Risk Assessment Toolkit: Chemical Hazards*[1]
- *Application of Risk Analysis to Food Standards Issues*, a Joint FAO/WHO Expert Consultation, Geneva, Switzerland, 13–17 March 1995[2].

As the process is incorporated into routine practice during acute public health events we hope that users will suggest improvements for this manual as well as provide additional case studies that will improve it and assist training.

Purpose of the manual

Rapid risk management of acute public health events reduces or prevents disease in affected populations and reduces negative social and economic consequences. Additional benefits include:

- defensible decision-making
- implementation of appropriate and timely control measures
- more effective operational communication
- more effective risk communication
- improved preparedness.

Defensible decision-making

Risk assessment takes into account and documents all relevant information available at the time of the assessment. This supports and directs decision-making and provides a record of the process including:

- which risks and control measures were assessed
- the methods used to assess them
- why they were considered important
- their order of priority.

---

1 http://www.who.int/ipcs/publications/methods/harmonization/toolkit.pdf

2 http://www.who.int/foodsafety/publications/micro/march1995/en/index.html

If documented consistently, risk assessment provides a record of the rationale for changes over the course of the event including the:

- assessed level of risk
- recommended control measures
- key decisions and actions.

Evaluation of the risk assessment – based on systematic documentation – provides an important means of identifying where improvements can be made and provides an evidence base for future risk assessments and responses to events.

Implementation of appropriate and timely control measures

The systematic approach to collecting and analyzing information about the hazard, exposures and context in which the event is occurring helps to:

- identify evidence-based control measures
- rank the suitability and feasibility of control measures
- ensure that control measures are proportional to the risk posed to public health.

In addition, because the risk is assessed repeatedly during an event, risk assessment offers authorities an opportunity to adapt control measures as new information becomes available.

More effective operational communication

Using a common risk terminology can greatly improve the operational communication between different levels of an organization and with other sectors and institutions involved in the assessment and response to the event.

More effective risk communication

The aim of public risk communication is to enable the target population to make informed decisions about recommended personal and community-based prevention and mitigation measures. Effective risk communication relies on the timely and transparent sharing of all relevant information, and the building of trust and empathy. A systematic approach to the assessment of acute public health events supports effective risk communication through the rapid dissemination of information and the identification of key prevention and mitigation measures.

Improved preparedness

Although the manual focuses primarily on the use of risk assessment during acute public health events the approach is equally applicable to preparedness activities, especially to seasonal and recurrent outbreaks (e.g. annual cholera outbreaks in Africa and the dengue season in the Americas and Asia). To aid preparedness planning, risk assessment can be used to identify at-risk areas or populations, rank preparedness activities, and engage key policy and operational partners.

How the manual was developed

A working group first met in Geneva, November, 2010 consisting of staff from WHO Country Offices, Regional Offices and Headquarters who were:

- responsible for event-based surveillance
- responsible for public-health event risk assessment across multiple hazards or specifically food safety or chemical hazards risk assessment
- experienced in leading outbreak responses
- experienced in delivering risk assessment training courses.

In addition, an animal health expert was involved in developing the manual and WHO risk communication and International Health Regulations (IHR) specialists were consulted.

A list of people who participated in the working group and subsequent telephone conferences is provided in Appendix 6.

Terminology

In the context of this manual, an acute public health event is any outbreak or rapidly evolving situation that may have negative consequences for human health and requires immediate assessment and action. The term includes events that have not yet led to disease in humans but have the potential to cause disease through exposure to infected or contaminated food, water, animals, manufactured products or environments.

Terms used to describe risk differ between disciplines. In this manual, risk is the likelihood of the occurrence and the likely magnitude of the consequences of an adverse event during a specified period. A comparison of 'risk' terms used in important sectors and disciplines relevant to public health is provided in Appendix 1.

There are historical reasons why different disciplines use different terms when considering risk. As this manual focuses on acute public health events, where multidisciplinary and multisectoral inputs into the risk assessment may be needed, the terms used are a practical compromise that have been proven to work across disciplines and are defined in Appendix 2.

The all-hazards approach and the International Health Regulations

An all-hazards approach has been used for many years in emergency and disaster management to describe natural, technological, or man-made events that require action to protect life, property, environment, and public health or safety, and to minimize social disruption.

It is applied to public health events that require an immediate response and are potentially caused by more than one hazard — including biological, chemical and radionuclear hazards, whether naturally occurring or as a result of an accident or deliberate release — and natural disasters such as fires, floods, other extreme weather events, volcanic eruptions, earthquakes and tsunamis.

This approach has been driven by the International Health Regulations (IHR), which were revised in 2005 to reflect growth in international travel and trade, emergence or re-emergence of international disease risks, and threats posed by chemicals, toxins and radiation.

The IHR requires all States Parties to the Regulations to develop a set of core capacities in surveillance and response covering any "illness or medical condition, irrespective of origin or source that presents or could present significant harm to humans".

Following a risk assessment, the Annex 2 decision instrument of the IHR are used by Member States to decide whether an acute public heath event requires formal notification to WHO. The effective use of Annex 2 depends on each national authority and its IHR National Focal Point (NFP) carrying out risk assessments on public health events occurring within their territories.

The IHR core capacity requirements for surveillance and response require Member States to develop a national (and, where possible, a sub-national) risk assessment capacity that is recognized as an integral part of the prevention, surveillance and response system. The structure and location of this capacity, which may be a dedicated team or embedded into the existing prevention, surveillance and response system, will be country-specific.

Despite differences in how Member States might structure and locate their risk assessment capacity, WHO and all Member States should use a consistent, structured approach to the risk assessment of acute public health events. Recommended steps in such a structured risk assessment are outlined in the following sections.

Detection and confirmation of a public health event

All Member States have surveillance systems that detect outbreaks of infectious diseases. As a result of the emphasis in the IHR on strengthening this core capacity, many Member States have expanded these systems to include public health events caused by other hazards. Surveillance systems detect public health events through:

- **Indicator-based surveillance:** The routine collection of pre-defined information about diseases[1] using case definitions (e.g. weekly surveillance of cases of acute flaccid paralysis). Predetermined outbreak thresholds are often set for alert and response.
- **Event-based surveillance:** The rapid collection of ad hoc information about acute public health events. Event-based surveillance uses a variety of official and unofficial information sources to detect clusters of cases with similar clinical signs and symptoms that may not match the presentation of readily identifiable diseases. Official sources include national authorities and other agencies such as the UN system. Unofficial sources include media reports, other unofficial public information (e.g. internet sites), reports from the public

Not all event reports and alerts generated through indicator and event-based surveillance systems describe real events, nor are all real events of public health importance. The number of 'false positives' (i.e. reported events that cannot be confirmed as real or when alert thresholds of indicator-based surveillance systems are exceeded but an outbreak does not result) depends on the objectives and design of the surveillance system and the organizational level at which the event is assessed.

Guidance should be developed to assist staff in the triage and assessment of newly detected events (see Box 1). Event triage uses the same principles for assessing the risk an event may pose to public health as the more formal risk assessment described in this manual.

Box 1: Example of guidance to surveillance staff for triaging incoming signals from surveillance activities

Question	Answer
Has the event been reported by an official source (e.g. local health-care centre or clinic, public health authorities, animal health workers)?	Yes ☐ No ☐
Has the event been reported by multiple independent sources (e.g. residents, news media, health-care workers, animal health staff)?	Yes ☐ No ☐
Does the event description include details about time, place and people involved (e.g. six people are sick and two died three days after attending a local celebration in community X)?	Yes ☐ No ☐
Is the clinical presentation of the cases described (e.g. a cluster of seven people admitted to hospital with atypical pneumonia, of whom two have died)?	Yes ☐ No ☐
Has a similar event been reported previously (e.g. with a similar presentation, affecting a similar population and geographical area, over the same time period)?	Yes ☐ No ☐

Incoming signals are more likely to describe real events if there are one or more 'yes' answers to the questions tabled above.

---

1   The term 'disease' is used in its broadest sense, including syndromes.

If the event is detected quickly, initial information may be limited and non-specific. The initial triage process focuses on assessing the credibility of the incoming signal(s) and whether the event described is a potential risk to public health that warrants investigation. The accuracy of the reporting of the event may be assessed at the same time. Confirmation of an event does not automatically mean that it presents a risk to public health. Some events may have little or no effect on human health or may be related to chronic diseases or issues that do not pose an acute public health risk. As a result, different actions may result from the initial risk assessment (see Table 1).

Table 1: Example of action taken as a result of triage and confirmation of an event

Outcome of triage and confirmation	Action
Reported event is proved to be a false rumour	Discard the event Risk communication and media communication about the event may be needed to address the public perception of risk (e.g. smallpox rumours)
Event is confirmed but is not an immediate public health risk	Monitor the event and undertake risk assessments as new information becomes available Risk communication and media communication about the event may be needed to address the public perception of risk
Event is confirmed and may be considered an immediate public health risk	Undertake a full risk assessment and state the level of confidence in the assessment Provide recommendations for decision-makers, including which actions should be taken and which should have the highest priority (e.g. recommended control measures, key communication messages) Undertake additional risk assessments and modify recommendations for decision-makers as new information becomes available. The actions taken as a result of the risk assessments will differ at different organizational levels

Introduction to risk assessment

Risk assessment is a systematic process for gathering, assessing and documenting information to assign a level of risk. It provides the basis for taking action to manage and reduce the negative consequences of acute public health risks (see Figure 1). The risk management cycle includes:

- risk assessment — hazard, exposure and context assessment and risk characterization in which the level of risk is assigned to the event
- identification of potential control measures — ranked by priority, taking into account likelihood of success, feasibility of implementation and unintended consequences for the affected population and society more broadly
- continuous monitoring and evaluation as the event unfolds
- effective ongoing communication to ensure that risk managers, other stakeholders and affected communities understand and support the control measures that are implemented
- an evaluation of lessons learned at the end of the response.

Figure 1: The risk management cycle

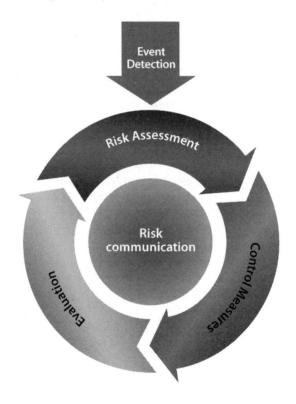

Steps in the risk assessment of public health events

Assembling the risk assessment team

After confirming that a reported event is real and may be considered an immediate public health risk, its public health importance must be determined. Depending on the quality and completeness of the information available to assess the risk, a risk assessment team may be assembled. Deciding on the disciplines that should make up the risk assessment team is a critical step that is often overlooked. Additional expertise (e.g. in toxicology, animal health, food safety or radiation protection) can be brought in at any time but may be needed at the beginning of the risk assessment if:

- the hazard is unknown
- the event is unlikely to be caused by an infectious agent
- an event is associated with disease or deaths in animals, and/or is otherwise identified as a suspected zoonosis
- the event is related to a food or product recall, known chemical accident, or radionuclear incident with or without reports of human disease.

Operational communication and risk communication are integral parts of risk management. At a minimum, links should be established between the risk assessment team and communication specialists. If possible, a communication specialist should be included in the risk assessment team. Ensuring that there is good communication between decision-makers and the affected population from the start of the process will increase the likelihood of effective implementation of control measures, especially those requiring behavioural change.

The knowledge and expertise of the team greatly influence the risk assessment. Local knowledge about the environment in which the event is occurring is a critical component of risk assessment. The level of risk of an acute public health event depends on the social, economic, environmental and political conditions in the affected area and the effectiveness of local health services (e.g. curative and public health services). For some hazards, the effectiveness of links between health services and other responsible sectors and agencies (e.g. with the animal health sector for zoonotic diseases) may also affect the risk and must be assessed.

Formulating risk questions

The risk assessment team should decide on the key questions to be answered. This helps to define the scope of the assessment and ensures that all the relevant information is collected. Clearly defined questions help identify priority activities to be conducted as part of the risk assessment. This may include literature reviews, epidemiological investigations, enhanced surveillance, consultation with disease experts, surveys and research.

A risk question is similar to a research question and typically focuses on:

- who is likely to be affected
- the likely exposure to a hazard
- when, why and how a population might be adversely affected by exposure to a hazard

The questions asked by the risk assessment team will be influenced by factors including:

- the population at risk
- the level at which the risk assessment is taking place – local, sub-national, national, international (e.g. cross-border), or global
- the technical and policy disciplines and agencies that are included in the risk assessment team and their collective experience with the type of event they are assessing (e.g. a well-characterized disease compared to a public health event of unknown cause (unknown etiology)
- the level of risk accepted by decision-makers, other stakeholders and society (i.e. the acceptable risk)
- the timing of the risk assessment during the course of the event
- the outcome of previous risk assessments carried out for the event and similar situations in the past
- the level of perceived external (e.g. international community) interest or awareness of the event.

The team should not try to answer all the possible risk questions at once. Instead, critical questions should be identified and ranked by priority for immediate response. Less time-critical questions can be addressed later or by other teams.

The main question asked during acute public health events is, 'what is the public health risk of the event' (i.e. what is the risk related to exposure to a particular hazard in a particular location, or to a particular population at a particular time)?

This question often leads to others, such as:

- What is the likelihood of exposure to the hazard if no action is taken?
- What are the consequences (type and magnitude) to public health if the event were to occur?

Risk questions may be framed as a series of scenarios, such as:

- What is the public health risk of the event in the current situation?
- What is the public health risk of spread to a major city?
- What is the public health risk of the event affecting more than one area (province/state, country)?

Other examples of risk questions in response to different scenarios are shown in Table 2.

Table 2: Examples of risk questions

Example of event report	Risk question
52 pigs died in two neighbouring farms over one to two days.	Could this be a risk to human health?
Clusters of people living with HIV/AIDS have suddenly become unresponsive to treatment.	Which hazards could cause this event? For example: • secondary infection • substandard medication (e.g. counterfeit drugs or loss of potency due to expired drugs) • drug resistance • availability of the drug (e.g. that leads to sharing medications or patients unable to access the medications) • patient adherence with treatment.
Pneumonia of unknown cause linked to deaths among health-care workers.	What is the likely cause (etiology) of the pneumonia? What are the possible public health consequences?
Two deaths and 16 suspected cases of cholera in a camp for internally displaced persons in a particular district.	What is the likelihood of further spread of cholera? What would be the consequences if this occurred?
Paediatric analgesic syrup formulated with diethylene glycol is identified after a cluster of deaths in children.	Is this product marketed abroad, either formally or informally? What would be the consequences if this occurred?
An outbreak of hand, foot and mouth disease (HFMD) in nursery school children in one of 14 regions in a country.	What would be the effect on disease transmission of implementing quarantine in the affected region? How would implementing quarantine measures affect disease transmission? What would be the consequences of implementing quarantine in the affected region?

Based on the characteristics of the event, the risk assessment team should decide how frequently the risk assessment should be updated. The team should also agree on the priority questions and decide the time needed to complete each assessment. The time available between assessments may help to direct the number and scope of risk questions considered.

Undertaking the risk assessment

The level of risk assigned to an event is based on the suspected (or known) hazard, the possible exposure to the hazard, and the context in which the event is occurring. Risk assessment includes three components — hazard, exposure, and context assessments. The outcome of these three assessments is used to characterize the overall level of risk (see Figure 2).

Figure 2: The risk assessment process

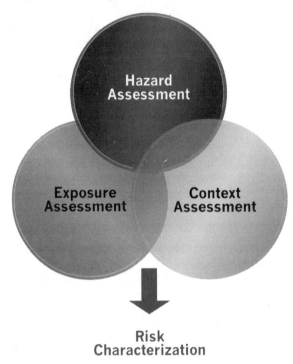

Completing a risk assessment is not always a sequential process with hazard, exposure and context usually assessed at the same time. Although each is assessed separately, there is overlap in the information required to assess each domain.

Hazard assessment

Hazard assessment is the identification of a hazard (or number of potential hazards) causing the event and of the associated adverse health effects.

Public health hazards can include biological, chemical, physical and radionuclear hazards. Hazard assessment includes:

- identifying the hazard(s) that could be causing the event
- reviewing key information about the potential hazard(s) (i.e. characterizing the hazard)
- ranking potential hazards when more than one is considered a possible cause of the event (equivalent to a differential diagnosis in clinical medicine).

When there is a laboratory confirmation of the causative agent or the event is easily characterized on clinical and epidemiological features, hazard identification can be straightforward. In such cases the hazard assessment would start with a known or strongly suspected hazard. However, in all other cases hazard assessment starts with listing possible causes based on the initial description of the event (e.g. the clinical and epidemiological features), known burden of disease in the affected community, and type and distribution of existing hazards (e.g. the number and location of chemical plants and the chemicals they use).

Medical practitioners, nurses, veterinarians and others working in clinical settings will be familiar with the importance of the differential diagnosis in the process of assessing a patient; hazard assessment is similar.

The less specific the information reported about an acute public health event, the broader the list of possible hazards becomes. However, as more information becomes available, the number of potential hazards is reduced and they can be ranked in order of the likelihood of being the cause.

The relative likelihood of a hazard can be determined by:

- the clinical features and natural history of the disease in humans or animals
- timing of the event and the speed with which the event evolves
- geographical area and settings affected
- the persons and populations affected

Table 3: Examples of questions to assess the likelihood of a specific hazard

Sample questions
• Does the suspected hazard (pathogen, toxin, contaminant etc.) cause the clinical signs and symptoms observed?
• Is the suspected hazard known to cause disease in humans or animals?
• Are the age group(s), sex or occupational group(s) affected typical for exposure to any hazards?
• Has the case(s) reported a history of recent travel?
• Is the time from presumed exposure to the onset of clinical signs and symptoms typical of a particular hazard or type of hazard?
• Is the severity of disease typical of a particular hazard or type of hazard?
• Does the disease respond to particular treatments (e.g. antibiotics)?
• Has the suspected hazard been diagnosed previously as the cause of disease at the same time of year, place or population?
• Have there been any associated or preceding events (e.g. disease or deaths in animals, food or product recalls, known accidental or deliberate releases of chemical, biological or radionuclear agents, similar events in neighbouring countries, etc.)?
• Do laboratory test results confirm a specific cause or are they consistent with a particular type of hazard?

Exposure assessment

Exposure assessment is the evaluation of the exposure of individuals and populations to likely hazards. The key output of the assessment is an estimate of the:

- number of people or group known or likely to have been exposed.
- number of exposed people or groups who are likely to be susceptible (i.e capable of getting a disease because they not immune)

Information required to answer these questions includes:

- modes of transmission (e.g. human-to-human transmission by droplet spread or direct contact transmission; animal-to-human transmission)
- dose–response (e.g. some infectious agents, toxins, chemicals)
- incubation period (known or suspected)
- case fatality rate (CFR)
- estimation of the potential for transmission (e.g. R0, the basic reproduction number).
- Vaccine status of the exposed population

For some hazards a dose–response relationship is an important determinant of the magnitude of exposure. Examples include the inhalation or ingestion of heavy metals such as lead, the number of salmonella bacteria ingested or the amount of a radionuclear isotope ingested or absorbed. For such hazards, in addition to assessing the exposure, the duration of exposure may also be important. With infectious diseases, differences in exposure can occur within households (e.g. measles), among close contacts (e.g. SARS) and other social networks (e.g. sexually transmitted diseases), in occupational risk groups (e.g. hepatitis B, Rift Valley fever, Q fever), and among travellers (e.g. malaria).

For vector-borne diseases (see Table 5) and other zoonoses, information about the vectors and their animal hosts is needed to assess exposure. This might include the species, distribution and density of vectors of disease, and the species, distribution and population density of animal hosts. The exposure assessment will provide an estimate of the likelihood that a particular area is vulnerable to the transmission of a zoonotic disease.

Context assessment

Context assessment is an evaluation of the environment in which the event is taking place. This may include the physical environment such as climate, vegetation, land use (e.g farming, industry) and water systems and sources as well as the health of the population (e.g. nutrition, disease burden and previous outbreaks), infrastructure (e.g. transport links, health care and public health infrastructure), cultural practices and beliefs.

Those who are trained in scientific disciplines, such as medicine, food safety and veterinary science, tend to approach risk assessment from a relatively narrow scientific perspective (e.g. of identifying the hazard) and may not consider other factors that affect risk.

Context assessment should consider all factors – social, technical and scientific, economic, environmental, ethical, and policy and political – that affect risk. These factors, summarized in the term STEEEP[1], can affect the level of risk by increasing or decreasing the likelihood of exposure or its consequences (Appendix 3).

Information (see Table 4) that helps to answer the following types of questions is a critical component of context assessment.

- What are the factors associated with the environment, health status, behaviours, social or cultural practices, health infrastructure and legal and policy frameworks that increase a population's vulnerability?
- Do any factors associated with the environment, health status, and social or cultural practices reduce the population's risk of exposure?
- What is the likelihood that all suspect cases can be identified?
- What is the availability and acceptability of effective preventive measures and of treatment or supportive therapies?

---

1 Some authors express STEEEP as 'PEST analysis' (omitting the 'E' for environmental and for ethical); others add an 'E' for environment and an 'L' for legal and speak of PESTLE; while others add an 'E' for ethics to this and speak of STEEPLE.

Table 4: Examples of the type of information that could be collected during a context assessment

Source	Type of information	Output from the assessment
Surveillance system	• Number of functioning reporting sites in the affected area • How suspected cases are identified	The likelihood that cases will be identified
Health-care infrastructure assessments or reports	• The number, location and quality of health-care facilities in the affected area • Health-seeking behaviour in the affected population	The likelihood that cases will seek and receive medical care that results in good clinical outcomes
Nutrition surveys from NGO or government reports	• Level of malnutrition in the affected area or among specific risk groups	The likelihood of severe disease
Information on animals and vectors	• Information on environmental conditions that might be favourable to population explosions of potential vectors of disease • Information on the number and distribution of potential animal hosts	The likelihood of outbreaks in humans or animals

The vector-borne disease, Japanese encephalitis, has been used to illustrate possible sources of information for assessment of the hazard, exposure and context (Table 5).

Table 5: Information sources used in assessing hazard, exposure and context of Japanese encephalitis

Characteristic being assessed		Information sources
Hazard assessment		
Viral factors	Genotypes	Published literature on research in humans and animals
	Neurovirulence	E.g. Database of nucleotide sequences (Genbank)
	Antigenicity	Reference laboratory data
	Proliferation	
Clinical factors	Clinical presentation	Medical records (ICD-10[1]), hospital-based sentinel surveillance systems, laboratory surveillance systems
	Clinical progression	
	Severity	
Exposure assessment		
Vector factors	Distribution, density and host preference of competent mosquito vectors	Published data (e.g. entomological surveys), vector control programme data (e.g. entomological surveillance systems including mosquito trapping, detection methods for JE virus in pooled mosquitoes, pesticide susceptibility data)
Host factors	Epidemiology of infection and disease in humans and other mammals (dead-end hosts)	Published research, including seroepidemiological studies and outbreak investigations
		Indicator-based and event-based surveillance systems in endemic and epidemic-prone areas (human and animal)
		Medical records, hospital-based sentinel surveillance systems, laboratory surveillance systems
		International event-based surveillance systems, including the media aggregators Biocaster, GIDEON, GPHIN, HealthMap, EMM MediSys, ProMED Mail, RSOE EDIS, among others.
		Surveys of permanent neurological impairment in endemic areas
		Official data and reports from WHO, FAO and OIE, other UN agencies, non-governmental organizations (e.g. PATH), foundations, charities (e.g. SciDevNet), national government websites of endemic countries. WHO sites reporting outbreaks include the Disease Outbreak News, Weekly Epidemiological Record and the password protected Event Information Site for IHR National Focal Points and ShareGOARN
		Participatory epidemiology systems
		Case reports of illness in returning travellers
	Distribution and susceptibility of amplifying hosts (pigs and aquatic birds)	Aquatic bird population, density and distribution of domesticated and feral pigs close to human populations
		Sentinel pig surveillance data
	Susceptibility (age, population immunity, vaccination status, protection from cross-reacting antibodies e.g. dengue)	Medical records and chart audits (ICD-10[1], acute neurological syndrome, etc.)

---

1   http://www.who.int/classifications/icd/en/

Table 5 *continued*

Characteristic being assessed		Information sources
CONTEXT ASSESSMENT		
Socio-economic factors	Size of population at risk Agriculture and livestock management	Vital statistics Demographic data including household income data (e.g. census) – access to personal protective equipment to prevent mosquito bites Maps of population density Economic analyses of pig farming in endemic areas
	Human behaviour	Surveys and studies on community awareness of Japanese encephalitis virus transmission; prevention and control; cultural practices regarding pig farming; acceptability and uptake of Japanese encephalitis vaccination etc. International transport (vectors, live pigs)
Ecological factors	Climate	Meteorological data (rainfall, temperature, wind) Modelling data on climate variability, climate change (e.g. World Meteorological Organization)
	Mosquito breeding sites	Entomological surveys; maps of standing water sources; town plans, reports on environmental engineering controls of breeding sites Remote sensing data of vegetation coverage, e.g. NASA Earth Observatory, Global Observing Systems Information Center (GOSIC)
	Amplifying bird hosts	Mapping data on bird migration patterns, seasonality and size of wetlands
	Feral pigs	Wildlife monitoring systems; data from culling programmes etc.
Program-matic factors	Strength of the health system (access to acute care services, intensive care units, diagnostic capacity, surveillance systems, Japanese encephalitis vaccination programme, vector control programme, financial and human resources, political support for control programmes including coordination with agriculture, livestock and wildlife sectors etc.)	National health indicator data Routine programmatic data, annual reports, programme evaluation reports etc. Vaccination coverage data (published and rapid assessment, public and private health-care facility data etc.)

Risk characterization

Once the risk assessment team has carried out the hazard, exposure and context assessments, a level of risk should be assigned. This process is called risk characterization. If there is no mathematical output from a quantitative model or comparison with a guidance value (e.g. in food safety risk assessments), the process is based on the expert opinion of the team.

A useful tool to assist the team is a risk matrix (Figures 3a and 3b) where estimates of the likelihood (see Table 6) are combined with estimates of the consequences (see Table 7).

As the majority of acute public health event risk assessments are qualitative, the categories used in the matrix are not based on numerical values but on broad descriptive definitions of likelihood and consequences (see Tables 6 and 7 and the legend for Figures 3a and 3b, which explains how to read the risk matrices).

When applying the matrix, the definitions of likelihood and consequence can be refined to fit with the national or sub-national context in each country.

Two styles of presenting the risk matrices are shown in Figures 3a and 3b. The choice of style of matrix depends on the team's preference; both styles serve as a visual tool to stimulate discussion and to help team members agree on a level of risk.

During discussions, team members should consider all types of consequences in addition to the expected morbidity, mortality, and direct long-term health consequences of the event (e.g. disability). This includes consideration of the STEEEP consequences (Appendix 3).

The risk matrix also helps to assess and document changes in risk before and after control measures are implemented. For some events, where information is limited and when the overall level of risk is obvious, the matrix may not be needed.

Figure 3a: A risk matrix showing clearly delimited boundaries between categories

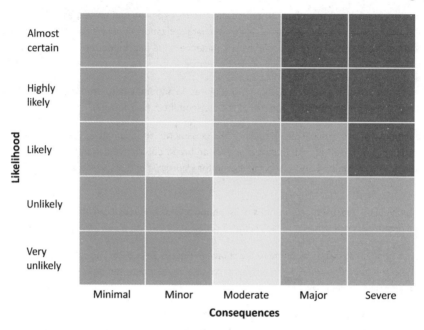

Figure 3b: A risk matrix without clearly delimited boundaries between categories

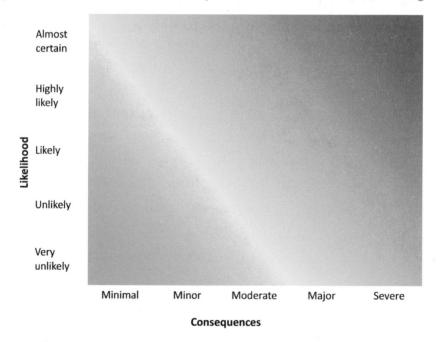

Table 6: How to read Figures 3a and 3b[1]

Level of overall risk	Actions
Low risk	Managed according to standard response protocols, routine control programmes and regulation (e.g. monitoring through routine surveillance systems)
Moderate risk	Roles and responsibility for the response must be specified. Specific monitoring or control measures required (e.g. enhanced surveillance, additional vaccination campaigns)
High risk	Senior management attention needed: there may be a need to establish command and control structures; a range of additional control measures will be required some of which may have significant consequences
Very high risk	Immediate response required even if the event is reported out of normal working hours. Immediate senior management attention needed (e.g. the command and control structure should be established within hours); the implementation of control measures with serious consequences is highly likely

Table 7: Estimates of likelihood definitions[1]

Level	Definition
Almost certain	Is expected to occur in most circumstances (e.g. probability of 95% or more)
Highly likely	Will probably occur in most circumstances (e.g. a probability of between 70% and 94%)
Likely	Will occur some of the time (e.g. a probability of between 30% and 69%)
Unlikely	Could occur some of the time (e.g. a probability of between 5% and 29%)
Very unlikely	Could occur under exceptional circumstances (e.g. a probability of less than 5%)

---

1   Adapted from WHO and FAO. *Risk Characterization of Microbiological Hazards in Food*. Microbiological Risk Assessment Series 17, World Health Organization and Food and Agriculture Organization, 1999. (http://www.who.int/foodsafety/publications/micro/MRA17.pdf).

Table 8: Estimates of consequences definitions[1]

Level	Consequences
Minimal	Limited impact on the affected population
	Little disruption to normal activities and services
	Routine responses are adequate and there is no need to implement additional control measures
	Few extra costs for authorities and stakeholders
Minor	Minor impact for a small population or at-risk group
	Limited disruption to normal activities and services
	A small number of additional control measures will be needed that require minimal resources
	Some increase in costs for authorities and stakeholders.
Moderate	Moderate impact as a large population or at-risk group is affected
	Moderate disruption to normal activities and services
	Some additional control measures will be needed and some of these require moderate resources to implement
	Moderate increase in costs for authorities and stakeholders
Major	Major impact for a small population or at-risk group
	Major disruption to normal activities and services
	A large number of additional control measures will be needed and some of these require significant resources to implement
	Significant increase in costs for authorities and stakeholders
Severe	Severe impact for a large population or at-risk group
	Severe disruption to normal activities and services
	A large number of additional control measures will be needed and most of these require significant resources to implement
	Serious increase in costs for authorities and stakeholders

---

1 Adapted from WHO and FAO. *Risk Characterization of Microbiological Hazards in Food.* Microbiological Risk Assessment Series 17, World Health Organization and Food and Agriculture Organization, 1999. (http://www.who.int/foodsafety/publications/micro/MRA17.pdf

Level of confidence in the risk assessment

It is important to document the risk assessment team's level of confidence[1] in the assessment and the reasons for any limitations. This will depend on the reliability, completeness and quality of the information used, and the underlying assumptions made with respect to the hazard, exposure and context.

The more evidence there is to inform the hazard, exposure and context assessments, the greater confidence the team can have in the results. The degree of confidence can be expressed using a descriptive scale that ranges from very low to very high.

Table 9 shows two scenarios that illustrate how levels of confidence can be estimated. Example A describes detailed information based on a variety of sources, including first-hand reports from clinicians, sources with local knowledge, historical records and peer-reviewed articles. A risk assessment based on these data would have a medium-to-high confidence score. In contrast, example B describes an event reported in a newspaper article that has not been confirmed by any other source. Any risk assessment based on this information alone would have a very low or low confidence score.

Table 9: Level of confidence in two risk assessments

Example A - High level of confidence	Example B - Low level of confidence
Hazard assessment based on: • a detailed clinical description of cases provided by hospital-based physicians • etiological (i.e. causative) agents known to have caused similar outbreaks in the previous two years • surveillance data	Hazard assessment based on: • a non-specific clinical description of cases reported in newspaper article • no historical data included in the report
Exposure assessment based on: • epidemiological investigation of the rapid response team • peer-reviewed articles and evidence from previous outbreaks	Exposure assessment based on: • the likely routes of transmission consistent with the clinical features reported in the media report (e.g. food- or water-borne transmission causing an acute disease with nausea, vomiting and diarrhoea)
Context assessment based on: • health-care system performance during previous outbreaks • external reviews • local sources: detailed information from local leaders and health authorities	Context assessment based on: • the knowledge and experience of a staff member in the risk assessment team

---

1   In some disciplines, the 'confidence' (or 'certainty') of an estimate is described as its reverse: its 'uncertainty' (see glossary of terms in Appendix 2).

Box 2: Example of risk characterization — severe respiratory disease

Event: A cluster of 22 cases of severe respiratory disease with seven deaths in country X were admitted to hospital over the past 17 days. The event is occurring 8 km from the border and cases have been reported from three villages by a local health-care worker (HCW). The area is the poorest in country X and health infrastructure is limited. Many of the health care facilities charge a consultation fee and consequently the local population self-medicates during mild illness. There are also strong beliefs that `strange diseases´ are caused by sorcery.

Risk question: What is the likelihood of further spread of severe cases of respiratory disease and what would be the consequences (type and magnitude) to public health if this were to occur?

Information used to assess the likelihood of further spread:

- cases are still being reported 17 days after the first known cases were detected
- the specific hazard and mode(s) of transmission have not been identified
- it is also likely that some cases are not being detected (e.g. mild cases are less likely to seek care from health services and are therefore not included in the official reports).

Therefore it is highly likely that further cases will occur if nothing is done.

Information used to assess the consequences of further spread:

- the disease has a high case fatality ratio (even when under-reporting is taken into account)
- the health-care system is poor and the ability to treat the cases is already limited; new admissions will further stress acute care services and lead to worse clinical outcomes for hospitalized patients
- negative economic and social impact of the cases and deaths in the affected communities
- there is potential for unrest in communities because of cultural beliefs that sorcery is causing the deaths

- the event is occurring in a border area and could affect the neighbouring country.

Therefore the consequences if further cases occur will be **severe.**

Using the risk matrix to combine the estimate of the likelihood and the estimate of consequences leads to an estimate of the overall risk; in this case, the overall level of risk is **high.**

The confidence in the risk assessment is **low-medium.**

Although the report is from a local HCW, the information is limited and it is not clear if the HCW has examined the suspect cases or is reporting a rumour.

Often at the start of a series of assessments, the risk assessment team will face the type of scenario outlined in Example B. The risk assessment will then rely on the opinion of the team and the interpretation of the limited information available.

It should be emphasized that a risk assessment with very low or low confidence does not indicate a poor risk assessment; rather it reflects the information available when the risk assessment was undertaken and the limitations of the data. It is important to include the confidence level in any conclusions and recommendations of a risk assessment (see Box 2).

Quantification in risk assessment

The degree of quantification that is possible in a risk assessment depends on factors such as the data available, how quickly the assessment is required and the complexity of the issues.

In some disciplines such as engineering, highly quantitative assessments are feasible. However, in the assessment of acute public health events a qualitative approach may be the only option, particularly early in an event when data are often limited or unavailable.

Even with biological risk assessments that might take much longer (e.g. in international trade, where major import risk analyses using large multidisciplinary teams might extend over several years), it is unlikely that reliable quantitative data are available for all steps in the risk assessment. In practice, many assessments use a mix of methods, using quantitative methods when numerical data are available and qualitative methods when they are not.

It should be emphasized that a quantitative risk assessment that uses poor data or inappropriate quantitative techniques can be far less scientific and defensible than a well-structured, more qualitative assessment. Appendix 4 provides some further information on issues related to quantification in risk assessment.

Control measures

The outcome of a risk assessment should be used to direct proportionate control measures that reflect the risk. The overall level of risk assigned to the event helps identify the urgency and extent of the control measures needed.

Both risk matrices can also be used to rank control measures according to their effectiveness. For example, they can be used to rank the likelihood that a control measure will prevent further spread or dissemination of a hazard (see Table 10) and the consequences of applying each control measure (see Table 11).

Table 10: The likelihood that a control measure will prevent further spread

Level	Definition
Almost certain	Is expected to prevent additional cases in most circumstances
Highly likely	Will probably prevent additional cases in most circumstances
Likely	Will prevent additional cases some of the time
Unlikely	Could prevent additional cases some of the time
Very unlikely	Could prevent additional cases under exceptional circumstances

Table 11: Consequences of implementing each control measure

Level	Definition
Minimal	Limited social impact
	No ethical considerations
	No or very little economic impact
	No or very little political impact
Minor	Minor social impact
	Limited ethical considerations
	Limited economic costs
	Some political impact
Moderate	Moderate social impact
	Some ethical considerations
	Moderate economic costs
	Moderate political impact
Major	Major social impact
	Significant ethical considerations
	Major economic costs
	Major political impact
Severe	Severe social impact
	Considerable ethical considerations
	Considerable economic costs
	Severe political impact

The risk assessment team should consider the STEEEP consequences of each control measure (Appendix 3). In doing so, the team should be careful to consider all aspects of STEEEP and not just one set of consequences (e.g. limiting the assessment to only the technical and scientific or biomedical effects of a control measure).

Assessing the likely effectiveness and consequences of control measures helps to ensure that they are appropriate to the risk of harm. This type of assessment can help the team convince decision-makers of the most appropriate set of control measures and to assist in deciding on the level of acceptable risk.

Generally, the control measures that are most likely to prevent spread or reduce adverse health and other STEEEP consequences and that have minor to moderate negative consequences are the most acceptable. However, in exceptional circumstances where the event is determined as high risk (i.e. almost certain to happen with serious consequences) and/or there is a low level of confidence (i.e. a high level of uncertainty) requiring a cautious or precautionary approach, control measures that may have only a limited chance of preventing additional cases or spread of the hazard may be acceptable.

Risk communication

Risk communication is an integral part of the risk management process and is described in more detail in Appendix 5. There are two equally important components to risk communication:

- Operational communication: The structured communication that organizations use to meet their work goals and strategic objectives, including coordination internally and with people and groups outside the organization. Operational communication occurs between the risk assessment team and relevant stakeholders (technical specialists and policy-makers at the relevant levels of government, other response agencies, the private sector etc.).
- Communication with the public: Communication to provide key findings from risk assessments at regular intervals. Regular communication helps to ensure that the public is informed of the nature and level of risks and the desired behavioural changes that can minimize them.

At the start of the risk assessment, the team should identify stakeholders. The communication strategy for each public health event should be agreed as soon as possible to ensure that there is two-way communication between the risk management team and stakeholders.

The strategy should include:

- how the team will provide regular feedback on the risk assessment, and in what format;
- clearly defined roles and responsibilities (e.g. focal points) for communications functions;
- how and in what format the information should be presented to stakeholders and the public.

Monitoring and evaluation

A risk assessment should be repeated as new information becomes available. It may also be repeated on a regular timetable (e.g. daily in the early stages of an event, perhaps driven by a Minister who agrees to provide an update to other Ministers or to the media at a specific time each day).

Each time a risk assessment is undertaken for an event it builds on the previous assessment. Each risk assessment (including the data and information available at the time it was undertaken) should be documented. Such documentation is an important part of monitoring and evaluation of the process.

Depending on the size and complexity of a public health event, many risk assessments may be needed to address new and different risk questions as the event progresses. For some events, different risk assessment teams may be required to work collaboratively to assemble the information for a composite picture of the risk (e.g. clinical severity, transmission dynamics, and control measures).

At the conclusion of the event, all of the risk assessments should be formally reviewed. The systematic analysis of well-documented risk assessments identifies where improvements can be made in the management of acute public health events.

APPENDIX 1:
Glossary of terms used in this manual

Acceptable risk	The level of risk that is tolerated or accepted. Hazards must be monitored to identify changes that could increase the level of risk. Defining acceptable risk should take into account informed consent and that 'acceptability' is likely to vary markedly between different stakeholders, populations and locations, and may be culturally specific.
Acute public health event	Any event that may have negative consequences for human health. The term includes events that have not yet lead to disease in humans but have the potential to cause human disease through exposure to infected or contaminated food, water, animals, manufactured products or environments.
Acute public health risk	The risk of an acute event resulting in negative consequences for public health.
Alert	The first notification that a public health event with adverse consequences may occur or may be occurring.
All-hazards approach	An approach to emergency management that takes into consideration all possible hazards — including biological, chemical, and radionuclear, hazards and natural disasters (e.g. fires, floods, other extreme weather events, volcanic eruptions, earthquakes and tsunamis).
Bias	The systematic deviation of results or inferences that distort the view of what is actually occurring.
Confidence	Confidence describes how sure the assessment team is of an estimate. It reflects what some disciplines call the certainty or uncertainty around an estimate. Even with perfect information (i.e. no 'uncertainty'), natural variation ('variability') still exists.
Confirmation	The process of seeking evidence to confirm the accuracy of information. Also, the conclusion of such a process (i.e. the state when information has been verified).
Consequences	The downstream effects that result from an action or condition that may be negative or positive. A negative public health consequence causes or contributes to ill health. Consequences may include social, technical and scientific, economic, environmental, ethical, or policy and political effects.
Context assessment	Assessing the environment in which the event is taking place.
Control measures	Interventions put into place to reduce the effect of a hazard on the exposed population.
Detection	Finding through systematic means.
Differential diagnosis	A systematic method for attaining a diagnosis through consideration of health and vital statistics according to age, sex, or some other factor.

Event-based surveillance	The organized and rapid capture of information about events that are a potential risk to public health.
Event report	A report that systematically documents the time, person(s) and place (including context) associated with an event.
Exposure assessment	The evaluation of the potential exposures of individuals and populations to the hazards identified in the hazard assessment.
False positive	A positive test result in an individual who does not have the disease for which the test was undertaken.
Hazard	An agent that has potential to cause adverse health effects in exposed populations.
Hazard assessment	Identification of the hazard (or list of potential hazards) causing the event and of the associated adverse health effects.
IHR	The International Health Regulations (2005).
IHR Contact Point	WHO points of contact for communication from Member State IHR National Focal Points.
IHR National Focal Point	The national agency or institution designated to liaise with, and be accessible to, WHO and Member States at all times for the purposes of giving effect to the IHR.
IHR reports	Reports that are generated from or to Member States to comply with IHR for assessment and notification of events that may constitute a public health emergency of international concern.
Indicator-based surveillance	The routine collection of pre-defined information about diseases[1] using case definitions (e.g. weekly surveillance of cases of acute flaccid paralysis). There are often predetermined outbreak thresholds for alert and response.
Infectious disease	A disease caused by a specific infectious agent or its toxic products that arises through transmission of that agent or its products from an infected person, animal, or reservoir to a susceptible host.
Likelihood	The probability of an event occurring.
NGO	Nongovernmental organization.
Outbreak	An epidemic limited to localized increase in the incidence of a disease.
Public health	Health programmes and services characterized by planning and intervening for better health in populations, including understanding and reducing the risks of disease, disability and death.
Precautionary approach	Principle 15 of the Rio Declaration produced at the UN Conference on Environment and Development (UNCED 1992) codified the 'precautionary approach' for the first time at the global level. This approach indicates that lack of scientific certainty is no reason to postpone action to avoid potentially serious or irreversible harm to the environment. This principle has been adopted by some other sectors, including public health. Note that the term is not used in other sectors (e.g. import risk analysis, in which one may adopt a cautious or conservative approach but not a 'precautionary' one).

---

1 The term 'disease' is used in its broadest sense, including syndromes.

Reliability	The degree of stability of results exhibited when a measurement is repeated under identical conditions.
Risk	The likelihood of the occurrence and the likely magnitude of the consequences of an adverse event during a specified period.
Risk assessment	A systematic process for gathering, assessing and documenting information to assign a level of risk. Risk assessment includes three components: hazard assessment, exposure assessment and context assessment.
Risk communication	Risk communication is the range of communication principles, activities and exchange of information required through the preparedness, response and recovery phases of a serious public health event between responsible authorities, partner organizations and communities at risk to encourage informed decision-making, positive behaviour change and the maintenance of trust.
Risk management	The process of weighing policy options in the light of a risk assessment and, if required, selecting and implementing appropriate intervention options, including regulatory measures. With respect to acute public health events, risk management is the process by which appropriate actions are taken to manage and reduce the negative consequences of acute public health risks.
Risk statement	A statement assigning the level of risk associated with the potential of an acute public health event. This statement should be accompanied by a statement of confidence in the level of risk.
Sensitivity	The proportion of actual positives that are correctly identified by a test (e.g. the percentage of sick people who are correctly identified as having a condition).
Syndrome	A group of clinical signs and symptoms that consistently occur together, or a condition characterized by a set of associated clinical signs and symptoms.
Triage	The process of determining if an event or alert detected by a surveillance system is a potential risk to public health and prioritizing it for action.
Vulnerability	A position of relative disadvantage. The extent to which an individual or population is unable or unlikely to prevent or respond to hazards.
Zoonosis (plural: zoonoses)	A disease transmissible between animals and humans.

APPENDIX 2: Definitions used by different sectors and disciplines

Terms used in food safety risk analysis

The Codex Alimentarius Commission (or 'Codex') defines three components for food safety risk analysis (see figure below):

- risk assessment
- risk management
- risk communication

The three components of the Codex approach to food safety risk analysis

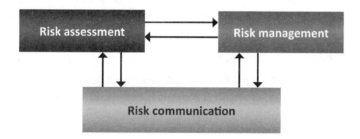

Codex uses the following definitions of terms in food safety risk analysis:

- *Hazard:* A biological, chemical or physical agent in, or condition of, food with the potential to cause an adverse health effect.
- *Risk:* A function of the probability of an adverse health effect and the severity of that effect, consequential to a hazard (or hazards) in food.
- *Risk analysis:* A process consisting of three components: risk assessment, risk management, and risk communication.
- *Risk assessment:* A scientifically based process consisting of the following steps: (i) hazard identification; (ii) hazard characterization; (iii) exposure assessment; and (iv) risk characterization.
- *Hazard identification:* The identification of biological, chemical, and physical agents capable of causing adverse health effects and which may be present in a particular food or group of foods.
- *Hazard characterization:* The qualitative and/or quantitative evaluation of the nature of the adverse health effects associated with biological, chemical and physical agents that may be present in food. For chemical agents, a dose–response assessment should be performed. For biological or physical agents, a dose–response assessment should be performed if the data are obtainable.

- *Exposure assessment:* The qualitative and/or quantitative evaluation of the likely intake of biological, chemical, and physical agents via food as well as exposures from other sources if relevant.
- *Risk characterization:* The qualitative and/or quantitative estimation, including attendant uncertainties, of the probability of occurrence and severity of known or potential adverse health effects in a given population based on hazard identification, hazard characterization and exposure assessment.
- *Risk management:* The process, distinct from risk assessment, of weighing policy alternatives in consultation with all interested parties, considering risk assessment and other factors relevant for the health protection of consumers and for the promotion of fair trade practices, and, if needed, selecting appropriate prevention and control options.
- *Risk communication:* The interactive exchange of information and opinions throughout the risk analysis process concerning hazards and risks, risk-related factors and risk perceptions, among risk assessors, risk managers, consumers, industry, the academic community and other interested parties, including the explanation of risk assessment findings and the basis of risk management decisions.

Terms used in import risk analysis

The Terrestrial Animal Health Code and the Aquatic Animal Health Code ('the Code(s)') of the World Organisation for Animal Health (OIE) describe four components in import risk analysis (see figure below):

- hazard identification
- risk assessment
- risk management
- risk communication

The four components of OIE's approach to import risk analysis

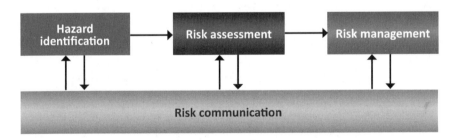

OIE uses the following definitions of terms in import risk analysis:

- *Hazard:* Any pathogenic agent that could produce adverse consequences on the importation of a commodity.
- *Risk:* The likelihood of the occurrence and the likely magnitude of the consequences of an adverse event to animal or human health in the importing country during a specified time period.

- *Risk analysis:* The process composed of hazard identification, risk assessment, risk management and risk communication.

- *Hazard identification:* The process of identifying the pathogenic agents that could potentially be introduced in the commodity considered for import.

- *Risk assessment:* The evaluation of the likelihood and the biological and economic consequences of entry, establishment or spread of a pathogenic agent within the territory of an importing country.

- *Risk management:* The process of identifying, selecting and implementing measures that can be applied to reduce the level of risk.

- *Risk communication:* Risk communication is the interactive exchange of information on risk among risk assessors, risk managers and other interested parties.

Further reading

Anderson K et al., eds. *The Economics of Quarantine and the SPS Agreement.* Centre for International Economic Studies, Adelaide, and AFFA Biosecurity Australia, Canberra, 2001.

Aven T. *Foundations of Risk Analysis: a knowledge and decision-oriented perspective.* John Wiley and Sons, Chichester, 2003.

Byrd DM and Cothern RC *Introduction to Risk Analysis: A systematic approach to science-based decision making.* Government Institutes, Rockville, Maryland, 2000.

Codex. *Risk Assessment Procedures used by the Codex Alimentarius Commission and its Subsidiary and Advisory Bodies.* Codex Alimentarius Commission, Food and Agriculture Organization, Geneva, 1993.

Covello VT and Merkhofer MW. *Risk Assessment Methods: approaches for assessing health and environmental risks,* Plenum Press, New York, 1993.

Flynn J et al., eds. *Risk, Media and Stigma: understanding public challenges to modern science and technology.* Earthscan. London, 2001.

Morgan MG and Henrion M. *Uncertainty: a guide to dealing with uncertainty in quantitative risk and policy analysis.* Cambridge University Press, Cambridge, 1992.

OIE. *Handbook on Import Risk Analysis for Animals and Animal Products. 2nd ed: Introduction and qualitative risk analysis.* World Organisation for Animal Health, Paris, 2010.

OIE. *Handbook on Import Risk Analysis for Animals and Animal Products. 2nd ed: Quantitative risk analysis.* World Organisation for Animal Health ,Paris, 2010.

OIE. *Aquatic Animal Health Code* (published online at http://www.oie.int/international-standard-setting/aquatic-code/access-online/). World Organisation for Animal Health, Paris, 2011.

OIE. *Terrestrial Animal Health Code.* (published online at http://www.oie.int/international-standard-setting/terrestrial-code/access-online/). World Organisation for Animal Health, Paris, 2011.

Renn O, ed. *Risk Governance: coping with uncertainty in a complex world.* Earthscan. London, 2008.

Robertson D and Kellow A, eds. *Globalization and the Environment: risk assessment and the WTO.* Edward Elgar, Cheltenham, United Kingdom, 2001.

Vose DJ. *Quantitative Risk Analysis: a guide to Monte Carlo modelling,* 2nd ed. John Wiley and Sons, Chichester, 2000.

APPENDIX 3: Examples of the STEEEP consequences of an acute public health event and associated control measures

Social

- Effects on individual cases placed in isolation, especially when hospitalized at a distance from their community
- Effects of restricted contact (e.g. for families visiting infected and seriously ill patients)
- Changes to important social or religious events (e.g. social distancing policies)
- Impact on lifestyle (e.g. changes to child care arrangements)
- Acceptability of the control measures by the affected community
- Social stigma from being a case of an infectious disease
- Psychological impacts

Technical and scientific

- Morbidity, mortality and long-term disability
- Effectiveness of control measures
- Ability to implement control measures in a timely manner
- Side effects of treatment or prophylaxis

Economic

- Direct financial costs for the preparedness and response agencies
- Direct financial costs of the response activities for the affected individual/families/communities (e.g. cost of treatments, health-care fees, loss of domestic and farmed animals)
- Indirect costs:
  - effect on individual and family ability to work (e.g. closure of schools, home isolation, hospitalization)
  - effect on household income
  - effect on the community income
  - effect on national economy
- The following should be considered at the local, national and international levels:
  - effect on travel and trade
  - effect on tourism

Environmental

- Negative effects of control measures on the natural environment (e.g. contamination or residues)
- Positive effects on the natural environment (e.g. simultaneous control of other diseases such as might occur with vector control)

Ethical

- Individual liberty (e.g. restricted movement)
- Unintended consequences (e.g. the removal of primary food sources for families when livestock is culled or contaminated crops destroyed and no alternative can be provided)
- Privacy
- Protection of the public from harm
- Use of unlicensed or unregistered drugs and vaccines
- Informed consent (i.e. that people understand what they are asked to accept or permit)
- Protection of communities and individuals from stigmatization (i.e. being regarded as unworthy or treated with disapproval)
- Proportionality (i.e. that control measures correspond to or reflect the risk)
- Duty to provide care (i.e. an obligation to provide safe, competent and ethical care to individuals or populations)
- Equity (i.e. being fair or impartial)
- Transparency (i.e. being open, obvious or evident)
- Unequal burden of risk (e.g. health-care workers, other first responders)

Policy and political

- Views of senior management in a response or supporting organization (e.g. compatibility with other programmes and policies)[1]
- Diversion of resources from other programmes and projects to support the response
- Views of the Minister of Health and other Ministers
- Views of Opposition parties
- Imminent elections and other politically charged situations
- Likely response of the media and key stakeholder groups
- Governments unwilling or incapable to respond effectively (e.g. political oppression or armed conflict; provision of access to care of internally displaced people or refugees)

---

1 These are sometimes called 'programmatic' risks.

APPENDIX 4: Quantification in risk assessment

The degree of quantification used in a risk assessment depends on factors such as the information available, how quickly the assessment is required and the complexity of the issues.

Some literature implies that there are two methods for risk assessment: 'qualitative' (using no or few numerical data) and 'quantitative' (using numerical data and computer modelling). However, even the most quantitative methods rely on qualitative, subjective judgement to formulate models and estimate parameters. Equally, even the most qualitative methods involve an ordering of risks and outcomes that is quantitative in the sense that they reflect the rules of the mathematics of probability and formal logic.

Structured formal risk assessment can use methods ranging from subjective reasoning based on descriptions of biological systems, to point-scoring systems, logical rules and Monte-Carlo simulation. Risk assessment can include methods that express inputs and results with varying degrees of numerical representation — that is, with varying degrees of quantification.

In some disciplines such as engineering, highly quantitative risk assessments are widely undertaken. Even in biological risk assessments that extend two or more years (e.g. in international trade, where major import risk analyses use large multidisciplinary teams), reliable quantitative data are unlikely to be available for all stages of the assessment. In practice, many assessments employ a mix of methods, using more quantitative methods when data are available and qualitative methods where they are not. In acute public health events a qualitative approach may be the only option, particularly early in an event when limited data are available.

Some methods use sensitivity analysis to determine if a particular parameter for which data are not available has a major effect on the overall risk. Such sensitivity analyses often show that there are only a few critical points in a pathway that have a significant effect on the overall risk. If good data are available on these points, the analyst can be confident that the assessment is robust. However, if good data are not available on these critical points, the analyst may use a less quantitative approach until appropriate research is conducted to obtain the data needed to undertake a more quantitative risk assessment.

Quantitative approaches are not necessarily better than qualitative approaches. A quantitative risk assessment that uses poor data or inappropriate techniques can be far less scientific and defensible than a more qualitative assessment. A well-structured and timely qualitative assessment is better than an incomplete and late attempt at a more 'quantitative' approach.

With respect to trade, all degrees of quantification are acceptable under the Agreement on the Application of Sanitary and Phytosanitary Measures (the SPS Agreement), and the World Trade Organization (WTO) recognises the validity of even the most qualitative risk assessments when they are appropriate to the circumstances.

Further reading:

Anderson K et al., eds. *The Economics of Quarantine and the SPS Agreement*. Centre for International Economic Studies, Adelaide, and AFFA Biosecurity Australia, Canberra, 2001.

Aven T. *Foundations of Risk Analysis: a knowledge and decision-oriented perspective*. John Wiley and Sons, Chichester, 2003.

Byrd DM and Cothern, RC. *Introduction to Risk Analysis: A systematic approach to science-based decision making*. Government Institutes, Rockville, Maryland, 2000.

Codex. *Risk Assessment Procedures used by the Codex Alimentarius Commission and its Subsidiary and Advisory Bodies*. Codex Alimentarius Commission, Food and Agriculture Organization, Geneva, 1993.

Covello, VT and Merkhofer MW. *Risk Assessment Methods: Approaches for assessing health and environmental risks*, Plenum Press, New York, 1993.

Morgan MG and Henrion M. *Uncertainty: a guide to dealing with uncertainty in quantitative risk and policy analysis*. Cambridge University Press, Cambridge, 1992.

OIE. *International Aquatic Animal Health Code* (published online at: http://www.oie.int/eng/normes/fcode/A_summry.htm). World Organisation for Animal Health, Paris, 2003.

OIE. *Terrestrial Animal Health Code* (published online at: http://www.oie.int/eng/normes/mcode/A_summry.htm). World Organisation for Animal Health, Paris, 2003.

OIE. *Handbook on Import Risk Analysis for Animals and Animal Products*, 2nd ed. *Volume 1: Introduction and qualitative risk analysis*. World Organisation for Animal Health, Paris, 2010.

OIE. *Handbook on Import Risk Analysis for Animals and Animal Products. Volume 2: Quantitative risk analysis*. World Organisation for Animal Health, Paris, 2004.

Robertson D and Kellow A, eds. *Globalization and the Environment: risk assessment and the WTO*. Edward Elgar, Cheltenham, United Kingdom, 2001.

Vose DJ. *Quantitative Risk Analysis: a guide to Monte Carlo modelling*, 2nd ed . John Wiley and Sons, Chichester, 2000.

APPENDIX 5: Risk communication

Risk communication is the range of communication principles, activities and exchange of information required through the preparedness, response and recovery phases of a serious public health event between responsible authorities, partner organizations and communities at risk to encourage informed decision-making, positive behaviour change and the maintenance of trust.

Risk communication is often listed last when it comes to risk management, which is not an accurate reflection of its importance. To be effective, risk communication needs to be planned and initiated early in a risk assessment and to continue as an iterative process throughout all phases of the assessment. If this does not happen, risk assessment is easily perceived as a process of expert risk assessors advising stakeholders of the result of their assessment and their proposed management strategies. This top-down approach implies that communication is largely one-way and ignores the need for consultation throughout the whole process. Poor risk communication can provoke outrage among stakeholders.

Problems in risk communication often arise because of the differences in world view between specialists and the public. These differences are reflected in the scientific and statistical language of specialists and the intuitive language of the public. The approaches are compared in the following table (adapted from Powell and Leiss, 1997)[1] .

Expert and public assessments of risk

'Expert' assessment of risk	'Public' assessment of risk
Scientific	Intuitive
Focused on 'acceptable risk'	Focused on safety ('no risk')
Changes with new information	Tends to be fixed
Compares risks	Focuses on discrete events
Uses population averages	Focuses on personal consequences
'A death is a death'	'It matters how we die'

Good risk communication seeks to 'translate' these languages to achieve cooperative understanding between all parties.

---

1   Powell D and Leiss W. *Mad Cows and Mother's Milk: the perils of poor risk communication.* McGill–Queen's University Press, Montreal, 1997.

Risk perception

Perceptions of risk by stakeholders and the public often align poorly with those held by expert assessors. A number of factors determine individual and group perceptions of risk. For example, analysis has shown that hazards perceived as unfamiliar or which provoke dread are assigned a higher risk than can be demonstrated statistically. Hazards with a low probability, which are regarded as having potentially catastrophic effects, are perceived as high risk and provoke strong public demands for government regulation and protection. Examples include a nuclear accident or the introduction of an unfamiliar disease that might be a zoonosis (e.g. ebola or nipah viruses), or the introduction of a known disease that might decimate native species. Risk assessors need to take account of these reactions in their communications with stakeholders and understand what provokes the feelings of these groups.

Even when good information is available on a hazard (i.e. where it is 'familiar'), the degree of trust given to the source of that information influences the perception of the risk. For example, surveys show that the public trust information from environmental groups or consumer organizations much more than that from government sources (and experts). Similarly, information provided by the media is trusted more than official government statements.

Lessons for good risk communication

The results of poor risk communication have been documented in a number of case studies such as the epidemic of bovine spongiform encephalopathy (BSE or 'mad cow disease'). Risk assessors, particularly those working on highly technical risk assessments, tend to focus on technical details. They may therefore be surprised to find their dedicated work on a risk assessment and their carefully reasoned recommendations for risk management provoke strong opposition. Leaving consideration of risk communication until late in the process, rather than involving stakeholders and the public early and often throughout the process, only increases the likelihood of such unfavourable reactions.

Powell and Leis (1997) defined 10 lessons in risk communication based on analysis of case studies of a range of animal health, food safety and public health issues:

- a vacuum in information on risk is a primary factor in the social amplification of risk
- regulators are responsible for effective risk communication
- industry is responsible for effective risk communication
- if you are responsible, act early and often
- there is always more to a risk issue than what the science says
- always put the science in a policy context
- 'educating the public' is no substitute for good risk communication practice
- banish 'no risk' messages
- risk messages should address directly the 'contest of opinion'
- communicating well has benefits for risk management.

APPENDIX 6: Contributors to the development of this manual

Dr Benido Impouma, Technical Officer, Epidemic and Pandemic Alert and Response Disease Prevention and Control Cluster, Regional Office for Africa, B.P.6, Brazzaville Republic of Congo

Dr Roberta Andraghetti, Advisor, International Health Regulations, Regional Office for the Americas, Pan American Sanitary Bureau, 525, 23rd Street, N.W. Washington, DC20037, United States of America

Dr Richard Brown, Regional Advisor, Department of Disease Surveillance and Epidemiology, World Health Organization, Regional Office for South-East Asia

Dr Graham Tallis, Medical Officer, Communicable Diseases Surveillance and Response Program Manager, World Health Organization, Country Office Indonesia

Dr Jukka Tapani Pukkila, Programme Manager, Alert and Response Operations, Division of Communicable Diseases, Health Security, & Environment, World Health Organization, Regional Office for Europe, 8, Scherfigsvej, DK-2100 Copenhagen, Denmark

Dr Shahin Huseynov, Technical Officer, World Health Organization, Country Office Uzbekistan

Dr Langoya Martin Opoka, Technical Officer, Disease Surveillance, Forecasting and Response, World Health Organization, Regional Office for the Eastern Mediterranean, Abdul Razzak Al Sanhouri Street, Nasr City, Cairo 1371, Egypt

Dr Ruth Foxwell, Epidemiologist, Emerging Disease Surveillance and Response, Division of Health Security and Emergencies, World Health Organization, Western Pacific Regional Office, 1000 Manila, Philippines

Dr Francette Dusan, Veterinary Epidemiologist, formally Communicable Disease Surveillance and Response, World Health Organisation, Lao PDR

Dr Mike J Nunn, Principal Scientist (Animal Biosecurity), Australian Government Department of Agriculture, Fisheries and Forestry, GPO Box 858, Canberra ACT 2601, Australia

Dr Angela Merianos, Project Leader, Risk Assessment and Decision Support, Alert and Response Operations, Department of Global Alert and Response, World Health Organization, Geneva, Switzerland

Amy Cawthorne, Epidemiologist, Risk Assessment and Decision Support, Alert and Response Operations/ Department of Global Alert and Response, World Health Organization, Geneva, Switzerland

Erika Garcia, Technical Officer, Risk Assessment and Decision Support , Alert and Response Operations, Department of Global Alert and Response, World Health Organization, Geneva, Switzerland

Dr Stephanie Williams, Medical Officer, formally Risk Assessment and Decision Support , Alert and Response Operations, Department of Global Alert and Response, World Health Organization, Geneva, Switzerland

Dr Andrea Ellis, Scientist, formally Risk Assessment and Management, Food Safety, Zoonoses and Foodborne Diseases, World Health Organization, Geneva, Switzerland

Dr Kersten Gutschmidt, Technical Officer, Evidence and Policy on Emerging EH Issues, World Health Organization, Geneva, Switzerland

Dr Danilo Lo Fo Wong, Coordinator, Antimicrobial Resistance, World Health Organization, Regional Office for Europe, 8, Scherfigsvej, DK-2100 Copenhagen, Denmark